Endorcements

"In the challenging world of auto-immune disease, Dr Ben's book offers a fresh perspective and hope for anyone looking to take charge of their health again."

-Dr. Jeremy Kerrigan

"When I met Dr. Ben I was in utter despair. I did not think I could hope again. I have many autoimmune complications such as arthritis, borderline celiac, histamine intolerance, gastroparesis and fibromyalgia. Yet in all of that Dr. Ben took the time with me and adjusted and re-adjusted his protocol again and again to fit my ailing body. 7 months later, I have a completely different life. I have hope now and I'm able to do a lot of things today. So working with Dr. Ben has been an extraordinary opportunity I never thought I'd have. I know, with absolute certainty, that reading the book you're holding in your hands today will also change your life as well."

-Ramsina S.

"I was dealing with seronegative rheumatoid arthritis and my hair was falling out. I was also not sleeping well and having difficulty losing weight. I followed the protocol and stayed as strict on it as I could for 6 weeks. My CRP inflammation level came down for a 5.2 to 2.2 and it really was a game changer. My hair stopped falling out. I have energy during the day and sleep soundly at night. My fingers do not feel as swollen and puffy as they did. This could possibly change your life because I know it changed mine."

-Deanna C.

"I've had MS since 2004. I had previously healed from it years ago on a whole food plant based diet. In 2019 it came back with inflammation and dizziness. In 2020 I decided to follow Dr. Ben's protocol. After 8 months I have no more pain and no more inflammation in my body! I hope you choose Dr. Ben's health protocol, it really works."

-Carol B.

"I used to have horrendous chronic sinus infections, I used to take 3-6 doses of medication a day. Since starting Dr. Ben's program they're pretty much non-existent. My digestive issues were so bad I used to spend a lot of time in the bathroom, but they're gone now. I pretty much got my life back. When I got my lab results back on my thyroid they were the best I'd gotten in my entire life, my TSH levels were almost zero which proves that this lifestyle change has been absolutely wonderful for me."

-Stephanie S.

CREATE HEALTH

HOW TO REVERSE AUTOIMMUNE DISEASE WITHOUT DRUGS OR THEIR SIDE EFFECTS

Benjamin Benulis, D.C.

JONES MEDIA PUBLISHING

DEDICATION

I want to dedicate this book to my late dog, Tuesday who gave me 14 years of love and support through both the best and worst of times of my life. I'm sorry we could not finish this book in your lifetime, but I know it would not have been possible without you.

Contents

FOREWORD

Autoimmune disease; genetics load the gun and environment pulls the trigger. Autoimmune diseases themselves result in the immune system attacking the body and if the disease won't kill you, the drugs used to treat the symptoms may. The options to reclaiming your health lie in your own decisions with your environment and food. Are you setting yourself up for success? Do you have a leader for your journey to freedom from autoimmune disease?

If you've picked up this book the chances are you're looking for a real healthy solution to your issues. Anything new is going to be uncomfortable to implement initially. Have you ever started a new job and had to learn a lot, or started a new workout routine and had growing pains in the beginning? As with anything else, the lifestyle changes necessary for resolution of your condition will cause some discomfort only to resolve with persistent application.

Dr. Benjamin Benulis, is a champion of health. He understands the processes that reverse complex autoimmune diseases and can result in newfound health. Having treated hundred of inpatients and outpatients alongside Dr. Benulis, I can assure you that he'll get straight to the point and not waste any time in getting down to the root of your issues. This book may save your life. I'm so excited to present my friend, Dr. Ben Benulis.

Dr. Peter Raisanen, NMD - IAHP certified naturopathic medical doctor, Medical Director of Men's Revival

Author's Preface

This book includes about a decade of experience as an auotimmune patient and as a healthcare practitioner: my own struggles with autoimmune disease; anecdotes and personal stories from many other sufferers, both friends and clients; clinical experience with patients; and voracious research, scrutinizing both books on health and the scientific literature.

While writing this book, I faced a problem early on: the vastness of the topic of autoimmune disease combined with how little science actually knew or could explain many of the phenomena. In fact, writing this book was put off for a long time to due to the Dunning-Kruger effect. This effect simply states that the more someone knows about a topic, the less confident they are in their assertions about said topic. Having studied this so intently for so long, I understand that there are massive gaps in the scientific understanding of what exactly autoimmune diseases are and what causes them. Additionally, even though we have scientific evidence to support that the therapeutic approaches I recommend here do in fact work, the actual mechanisms of action—*why* they work—are not well understood.

Acknowledgments

Trying to acknowledge everyone who has helped me out on my journey is an arduous task as many people have helped in big and small ways over the years. I am sure I will forget some people and for that I apologize. First off, my deepest gratitude goes to all the people who encouraged me to change careers when I first got the idea. Without them, so many things would not have happened: Dr. Nick Askey, Mike "Bonebreaker" Crockett, and Dr. Linda Carney. I owe a debt of gratitude to many teachers, mentors who have had an influence on me along the way: Dr. Robert Lockhart, Dr. Chris George, Dr. Alan Goldhamer, and Dr. Michael Soloman. My work is heavily influenced by the writings and works of many who have come before me but most notably: Dr. Doug Graham, Dr. Herbert Shelton, Dr. Candace Pert, Dr. T. Colin Campbell, Dr. Donald Esptein and Dr. Stephen Covey to name a few. I also owe a debt of gratitude to the coaches in various capacities who encouraged me along the way with writing this book: Justin Feldman, John Joseph McGowan, and Dr. Josh Sharpe. I also want to thank people who encouraged me to write a book and helped out with the early stages: Laurie Masters and Jessica Smothermon. I'd also like to thank several other doctors whom I consider col-

5

leagues who have been there to answer questions or think through tough problems over the years: Dr. Peter Raisanen, Dr. Kevin Pecca, Dr. Daniel Chong, Dr. Csilla Veress, Dr. Sarah Kashdan, Dr. Jeremy Kerrigan and Dr. Ben Karas. Lastly I want to thank my family who despite many times not understanding what I was doing, supporting me regardless.

INTRODUCTION: MY STORY

> You never change things by fighting the existing reality. To change something, build a new model that makes the existing model obsolete
>
> **—R. Buckminster Fuller**

They say that life is what happens to you when you're busy making other plans. They could say the same thing about autoimmune disease. I was certainly minding my own business doing other things. I was almost a decade deep in my first career in the semiconductor industry, working for a company that made tiny microchips that went into everything from TVs and computers to cars and microwaves.

At one point I started to notice mild annoyances that would later snowball into full blown severe symptoms. In the beginning I noticed that my energy was dipping. I became much more dependent on caffeine than I already was. My cognitive abilities started to slip. I went from being fairly good at my job to having a difficult time keeping up with everything that was going on. I also started to notice discomfort after some meals, like what I ate disagreed with me, even though I had never experienced that before.

Over the course of about eight to nine months these symp-toms increased to where it really started to interfere with my life. The fatigue got to where I was putting down two to three energy drinks a day just to get through the workday. I would be exhausted and sleep most of the weekend. The brain fog got to where my boss called me to his office to ask what was going on. Why was my performance at work slipping so bad when I had previously been a top performer? He said that if I didn't get my act together, I was in danger of failing my per-formance review at year-end and losing my job. I developed a chronic pain that just seemed to manifest as this constant muscle soreness that moved around to different parts of my body but never really went away. I also started to get ecze-ma-type rashes on my fingers and hands the likes of which I had never seen before. The rashes would come on strong for four to five days, slowly dissipate, then come raging back. They'd wax and wane in their severity but never fully go away. Also, my digestion became unbearably bad. It seemed that every full meal I ate, I was lying down in pain for almost an hour, clutching my sides. I had terrible gas, constipation, and bloating as well. My digestion was a mess.

It finally got to the point where I realized I should prob-ably go to the doctor. I was very unprepared for how disap-pointing and troubling an experience this would be. I report-ed my symptoms to my primary care provider, who told me I should take over the counter medication for my stomach troubles, and "try and get some more rest." I asked him to do bloodwork just to see what was wrong, he reluctantly agreed.

The follow-up visit was extremely troubling. He said, "All your blood work looks normal." I told him I still had symptoms; he said there was nothing he could do, except refer me to a specialist. To this day, I don't know what this specialist actually specialized in. But he looked at my bloodwork, shrugged his shoulders and said, "Yeah, everything looks normal. I don't know what to tell you, you're fine." I was *definitely not* fine.

During this time I really felt like my life was closing in on me. Not only was my physical health failing, but my job was on the line because I couldn't handle my workload any more. My social life suffered severely too. I was always too tired and too sick to hang out with friends. Additionally, my wife at the time pretty much didn't take me seriously that I was actually sick. She resented the fact that I didn't want to do things, always felt ill after meals and was just generally no fun to be around. She thought I was just being dramatic. It really strained our relationship. I started to get extremely depressed, because not only was I losing my physical health, I was in danger of losing my job, my relationship, and so many things that mattered to me.

I finally, reluctantly decided to get a food allergy test. Just to see if what I was eating was affecting me. So they drew some vials of blood and told me to wait two weeks for the results to come back from the lab.

During this waiting period I became intensely curious. What if I, in fact, did have a food allergy? It had seemed so preposterous at first. If I had a food allergy, wouldn't I know by now? Isn't that something you're born with? Could it really be that you develop it later in life? It seemed odd to me. But now, knowing what I know, it's possible, and it happens *all* the time.

I started calling the office, seeing if they got the results back from the lab. This was uncharacteristic of me; I'm usually not the type to be pesky. But I was dying of curiosity. I was calling the office every day to see if they got the results back. Finally, they called me on a Friday afternoon. As I recall, it went something like this:

"Hi, Ben, this is Dr. So-and-So down at such-and-such. We got your results back from the lab. I know you've been wanting to hear the results on these so I wanted to get back before the weekend. So the results came back and you did test positive for sensitivities to several foods, so I wanted to go over them with you.

"On a scale of 1 to 7 [Where do they come up with these numbers?] you tested a 7 for the following foods." He then went on to rattle off a litany of basically everything I was eating: "gluten, dairy, soy, casein, brewer's yeast, wheat, lactose . . ." The list went on.

So I said to the doctor, "Well, okay, so what kind of medication are you going to put me on?" In retrospect that sounds like the most ludicrous question to ask, but at the time, that is the level of consciousness where I was operating. My understanding of the medical model was that they test and examine you, come up with a diagnosis and then give you medicine to "cure" the condition. I thought they knew everything and had a 100 percent foolproof solution for every problem.

"Oh no," he said. "There's no medicine for this condition, you have to cut these foods out of your diet." Whoa, whoa, wait what? It was like there was a giant record scratch. I started thinking . . . I can't cut these foods out of my diet. They're in everything I eat. Without them, what am I going to eat? Gluten-free air sandwiches?

So here I was, left to fend for myself and figure this out on my own. In retrospect, it's funny that the doctor gave me very detailed information on what I shouldn't or couldn't eat, but absolutely no information on what I *should* eat. This was the medical model directly at work. Determine what is wrong and explain it to the patient, but don't look at anything that works or how to encourage more of what works.

So I did what any reasonable person would do. I went to the "health food" store and got the same stuff I was eating before, just without the gluten, dairy, soy, or flavor. Sounds reasonable enough, right? I was buying the Amy's vegan gluten-free macaroni and cheese. It costs way more money, and it tastes like cardboard. So far, getting healthy really sucked. I mean all I ate was microwave and packaged foods before, so I was just getting the same stuff without the allergens. Here's a surprise: I wasn't actually feeling all that much better other than my stomach was maybe 20 percent less agitated.

Frustrated with lack of results, lack of taste, and spending so much more on food, I was determined to figure something else. I had always identified as lazy when it came to cooking. I didn't want to learn how to cook. I needed simple and easy. So I figured out a way I could do this and still eat

11

even healthier. I would just start making smoothies, because smoothies are kind of like microwave food right? A blender operates similar to a microwave in a lot of ways. You open it up, throw the food in, push a button, and a minute later, your food is ready. All I needed to do was apply this microwave philosophy to smoothies right?

It started off somewhat successful. I just took whatever fruits and vegetables were in the fridge, threw them in the blender and hoped for the best. Some of the smoothies tasted great, some were OK, and some were just completely unpalatable. I realized that it needed some work. That was when I got the genius idea to look up smoothie recipes.

When I typed "smoothie recipes" into the search bar on YouTube, I was in no way prepared for the rabbit hole I was about to fall into. All I wanted were some recipes to make my smoothies taste better. What I ended up getting was a mind-blowing education in plant-based eating, raw foods, veganism, spirituality, biology, human physiology, philosophy, and many other subjects.

I started doing bigger smoothies. I started doing smoothies as entire meals, sometimes more than once a day. Within a month or two, I had bought a juicer as well. I became obsessed . . . and with good reason. I immediately started feeling much better. My chronic pain vanished in a matter of days. My digestion—as long as I was staying on program— was drastically improved. The brain fog lifted. My energy levels slowly increased. The rash on my hands began to decrease significantly in severity.

Within about two to three months I had undergone a massive transformation right before my own eyes. All I had really wanted was to eat food that wouldn't blow up my stomach. But what I got was an entirely new lease on life. My symptoms were 80–90 percent better and as a side effect, I was feeling the most positive, upbeat, and happy I had felt in a very long time.

Two things happened as a direct result. Number one, I became obnoxiously evangelical about what I was doing. I felt so good, I felt it was my duty to tell everyone I knew. Almost no one wanted to hear it. Everyone thought I was just being stupid or obnoxious.

Number two, with all this new energy, I upped my fitness game big-time. I had been working out at a personal-training studio where they track all your numbers. At this point, my trainer asked me what was going on? My lifts were increasing at a rapid rate, and I had the best strength-to-weight ratio of anyone who trained there. What was I doing?

The answered was severely bemusing: "Oh, I'm just eating healthier, a lot more fruits and vegetables, smoothies and juices. I cut out dairy and gluten, and a bunch of other junk." So then I was asked about my meat intake (I wasn't eating that either) and then scolded that I wasn't getting enough protein. "But you just said I have the best lifts and the best strength-to-weight ratio of anyone who trains here! Doesn't that mean what I'm doing is working?" They didn't want to hear it. But my numbers proved otherwise, so arguing seemed pretty much pointless. Besides, I was paying them good money to train there.

I started getting into endurance racing because I just needed the challenge. I started knocking off Tough Mudder races and half-marathons just because I could. I really felt I was on a mission to see what my body could do. I had gone well beyond just making my symptoms go away, I had reached an entirely new level of health that I didn't even know existed.

Philosophical Framework

I want to begin this work by establishing the lens through which I'll be looking at things. I think this is important, because if our perspective is faulty, we will likely never find the answers we seek. And I think a great deal of our inability to find an effective solution for autoimmune disease stems around the fact that we are looking at it through the wrong lens. Allow me to explain:

Create Health vs. Fighting Disease

Have you ever noticed that we never win most of the "wars" we declare on various enemies? We declared a war on cancer in the 1970s. Cancer is now the second leading cause of death, and poised to eventually become number one. Cancer is winning the war. We declared a war on drugs in the 1980s. Americans are taking more prescription drugs now than ever before. The opioid problem is so big it's been called an *epidemic*. The drugs are winning the war on drugs. We declared a war on terror in 2001. We still have plenty of terror. Trying to fight things you're opposed to rarely goes well. You may have heard the saying "What you resist, persists."

If you are so focused on the problem, you will never find a solution. Albert Einstein said, "We cannot solve our problems with the same thinking we used when we created them." We are so focused on what the problem is, and how to resist it, we cannot open our minds to any alternative. We cannot think a level higher as to what created the problem, and solve that.

For example, for most people who deal with addiction to drugs or alcohol, the substance is not really the problem. The substance is an attempt to solve a bigger problem, such as past trauma, low self-esteem, or lack of connection.

Fighting disease will only lead to more confusion and more disease. We must instead think at a higher level. Instead of focusing on destroying what we don't want, a higher level perspective would be to create what we *do* want.

So instead of trying to focus on *fighting disease*, I want this book to teach you to focus instead on *creating health*. This is such a huge shift in perspective that most people find it preposterous: that you could somehow make disease obsolete by just creating enough health.

The sad fact is that people in the twenty-first century are so grossly unhealthy and chronic disease is so normalized that they have no frame of reference for what it truly means to be healthy. So of course this idea will sound preposterous.

But let's build this assertion up from fundamentals. On some level we understand that the body has the ability to heal itself. We know that if we cut our finger, eventually it will heal. We also know that if we rub dirt in the cut, or pick at the scab as it forms, the healing process will be impeded until we leave it alone. Once we stop interfering with it, the healing can continue. If we put a bandage over the cut, it heals even faster.

But have you ever taken a bandage off of a cut, seen the healed finger underneath, and gone, "Wow, this bandage healed me! So amazing! Thank you bandage for healing me!" No, of course not, that's preposterous. The bandage has no healing properties per se. It did not actually heal you.

What did the bandage do? It *facilitated* the healing process. It did not do any healing itself. But what it did do was help provide the body with the optimum conditions *to heal itself*. Because the body could have healed the cut on its own, just slower. The bandage kept out any dirt or infectious agents that would have interfered with healing, but it performed no healing of its own.

This may seem obvious, but it's a very important nuanced point. Yes, the body heals itself, but only to the degree that we remove the interference and provide the optimum circumstances for this self-healing to occur.

The leap I am asking the reader to make is that this principle applies to almost any chronic disease. If we can provide the absolute optimum conditions for health, the body is capable of performing what many perceive as "miracles," healing from diseases that modern medicine considers "incurable." But the only reason this seems so is that the conditions we provide to our body in twenty-first-century Western society are so perverse that chronic disease is a normalized, common, expected outcome of everyday life.

Another analogy I love is the story of the garden, as told by the late Dr. Alec Burton, a pioneer in the field of natural health.

Once upon a time there was a man who purchased a very run-down garden in Scotland. The lot that he purchased was total wilderness. Absolutely rough and ruddy. But this man, he worked diligently for many weeks, for many months until it became a garden that was the most beautiful in the whole neighborhood . . . and people used to come from miles around to see this beautiful garden.

One day, the local priest came along and he saw the man working in his garden. He said to the man

"It's a beautiful garden you have here."

And the man said, "Yes, and I've done it all myself!"

"No," said the priest. "Not without the help of the Lord!"

He said, "Alright with the help of the Lord, yes, but you should have seen it when he was doing it by himself!"

A funny story yes, but what is the lesson here? The man was not providing the growth of the plants. He was not providing the essence of life. He was merely manipulating the factors of the environment, whereas the plants had the inherent ability to grow, to develop, and to prosper into the beautiful garden.

As with our own health, we cannot provide the actual spark of life. Outside forces cannot heal anything per se. Outside forces can only affect the outside circumstances to be advantageous or disadvantageous to the body's ability to heal itself.

For something like autoimmune disease where the body is severely chronically ill, we must provide the absolutely optimum circumstances for self-healing. The problem is that these circumstances are not something that many people are aware of, and even fewer are willing to put in the consistent work to create them. But if your goal is optimal health and you are determined to get there, you will do what it takes and put in the work, no matter how difficult it may seem. That is what I intend to teach you in this book.

So what are the optimum conditions to provide the body to ensure the best chance at healing itself? What are the fundamental building blocks for *creating health*?

- Eating a diet of the most optimal foods for the human organism, fresh fruits, and vegetables.
- Getting sufficient rest and sleep. These are the times when the body is able to put the most work toward healing itself.
- Regular movement and exercise. Fitness is a prerequisite of health. You can certainly be fit but not healthy, but you cannot be healthy without being fit.

- Stress-management strategies like meditation, breathwork, journaling, tapping, and other modalities that affect the overall tone of the nervous system.
- Strong relationships and social support. These are extremely important to our overall well-being.

These are the fundamentals. You could put this book down and have everything you need to know right here. But I will spend the rest of the book going in depth on this so you can walk away empowered, with a plan to make it happen for you.

If this approach sounds vastly oversimplified to you, understand that you are not alone. In twenty-first-century Western society, we have been conditioned to believe that complex problems *must* have a complex solution—and that such a simple solution simply cannot be.

When I began to adopt these principles of creating health myself in 2010, I was dumbfounded at how quickly my body began to heal itself. I witnessed my body completely transform from chronically ill to vibrantly well in a mere matter of weeks to months. Had it not happened to me firsthand, I would have never believed it. That experience completely transformed not only my body, but my entire paradigm of how health and disease actually worked. You can read about it in this book, and you can read the anecdotal stories of others, but until you actually experience it for yourself, you will never truly know.

What I want to get into next is explaining this perspective more in depth, and why the current fighting-disease model simply cannot help us solve most of the health issues we face today, both individually and as a society.

Medical Model vs. Alternative Medical Model vs. Health Model

Most of the modern world operates on what is called the *medical model*. For the first twenty-eight or so years of my life, this was how I viewed the concepts of health and disease. My concept was that if you were well, that was pretty much due to good fortune. If by bad luck you got sick, your course of action was to go to a doctor, who would examine and diagnose you with a disease, then prescribe you a medication to cure said disease. This is a very quid-pro-quo (Latin for *this for that*) model, wherein each disease is a discrete entity and each disease has a corresponding cure that only a doctor knows, because they were taught about all the diseases and all the cures in medical school. So it was quite the shock to my system when I went to the doctor and they could neither cure me nor diagnose me. Not only could they not diagnose me, they had a great deal of difficulty even acknowledging that I wasn't well. Since my set of symptoms did not seem to fall into any of the boxes they had learned about, few were willing to try to put a square peg through a round hole.

What the medical model essentially asserts is that the forces, influences, substances, and conditions that get a sick person well are different than the forces, influences, substances, and conditions that keep a well person well. For example, you only take drugs if you are sick. Once you get well, you should stop taking the drugs. In fact, if you take drugs when you're well, there's a good chance the drugs will make you sick. That's why we have prescriptions. Because if you take the drug when you're not sick, or you take the wrong drug, they can make you sick.

Rising in popularity in recent years is what's called the *alternative medical model*. While it may seem very different initially, it is actually very similar to the medical model. Alternative medical practitioners subscribe to the idea that traditional drugs and surgeries are often dangerous and/or ineffective, so they seek to provide alternatives to such practices. Instead of providing prescription drugs to suppress symptoms of disease, they provide supplements, herbs, oils, or other "natural remedies." It is still what's called the *outside-in approach*. It is still predicated on the idea that the human body is inherently faulty and needs the help of outside substances or forces to get well when it is sick. So while it comprehends the toxicity and the failures of the modern medical system, it fails to comprehend some simple, but very nuanced ways in which the human body-mind actually works. It is still the idea that the forces, influences, substances, and conditions that get a sick person well are different than the forces, influences, substances, and conditions that keep a well person well.

For example, in the alternative medical model, people will eschew traditional pharmaceutical antibiotics but be happy to use various naturally occurring substances, such as such as essential oils or colloidal silver, as antibiotics, instead.

They understand that pharmaceutical antibiotics may have side effects or destroy healthy bacteria in our system but fail to comprehend that a "natural" antibiotic could do the very same thing. They are still very much ingrained in this quid-pro-quo model of approaching health and disease; they have just applied it to a separate set of remedies.

The *health model* is very different from both the medical model and the alternative medical model. It states that the forces, influences, substances, and conditions that get a sick person well, are the *same* as the forces, influences, substances, and conditions that keep a well person well. Proper diet, nutrition, adequate sleep, adequate exercise, relationships, stress-mitigation practices: these are the forces, influences, substances, and conditions that *create health*. And they work whether you are sick or you are well. There is no danger of continuing with any of these once you transition from sick to well. They worked, keep doing them! This model understands and honors the body's miraculous ability to heal itself when given the proper conditions. If you read the original writings of founders of fields like naturopathy and chiropractic, they are based on these principles: that health results from healthy living, that the body has the ability to heal itself *when the interference is removed*, and that health, not disease, is the default state of being.

This model honors the body's natural ability to heal itself. It recognizes that our body is sovereign, capable, and miraculous given the proper conditions. The body does not need a cure or a miracle; the body performs the miracle, under the sole caveat that you remove the interference and provide it the conditions to do so.

Life would kind of be easier if the medical model or the alternative medical model worked right? If they did, you wouldn't need to take any responsibility for your own health because your actions would have no influence over it. You could just go to someone else when your body stopped functioning properly and they could "fix" you. Unfortunately it doesn't work that way. But that's a good thing too. It means that for the most part, your health is in your own hands. You have control over your destiny. Your actions shape your health. So act accordingly. The health model is a double-edged sword that grants you both the responsibility and the opportunity for amazing health, should you be willing to do what it takes to achieve it.

What if Car Insurance Worked Like Health Insurance?

I want to speak about the healthcare system in the modern world. Because it has failed us both in delivering health and by misleading us into grossly misunderstanding how health and disease actually work.

The gross dysfunction of the American healthcare system is probably something I will eventually write an entire book on. But I think it is vital for you to fundamentally understand how it works.

Currently, our healthcare system prefers drugs and surgery to treat diseases of diet and lifestyle. High blood pressure, type 2 diabetes, heart disease, and autoimmunity are treated with drugs and surgery. Even though these are diseases that people behaved their way into with their diets and their lifestyles, we are trying to medicate them out of it. As you know by now, it's a strategy that doesn't work very well. And it does not make a lot of logical sense that your health insurance would be fine with your causing your disease with your lifestyle and then paying you to see doctors to try to treat it with drugs.

Imagine if car insurance worked that way. Currently, car insurance will cover damage to your car after getting into an accident. If you have the right coverage, it will cover you even if the accident is your fault. But what won't the car insurance cover? Well, it won't cover changing the oil, that's on you. It won't cover routine maintenance, that's on you. If something breaks down mechanically from just normal wear and tear, it won't cover that either. If you're grossly negligent and don't change the oil, neglect the brakes squeaking, or let other maintenance slide and the car experiences worse problems . . . well, insurance definitely isn't covering that either.

But now think about your health. You can neglect it, harm it, run it into the ground. Smoke, drink, do drugs, eat horrible fast food, and so on, causing yourself all kinds of lifestyle disease—and guess what?—your insurance still has to cover it. Can you imagine if car insurance worked the same way? That people could be absolutely negligent idiots running their cars into the ground and their insurance would still pay? All the people who did the regular routine maintenance and repairs to keep their cars running well would be outraged that their premiums went up because of the people who are that negligent! They wouldn't stand for it! The free market would probably cause new insurance companies to sprout up who didn't pay for that kind of thing so that they could keep their premiums low. Honestly, I wish that would happen in the health insurance industry.

But that is why health insurance costs are so high. Because someone gave themselves type 2 diabetes with hamburgers and hotdogs. And instead of doctors putting them on fruits and vegetables, they're put on metformin and insulin, their toes are amputated, their heart vessels are stented or bypassed with surgery, their vision problems are treated by an eye doctor, and every downstream consequence of that disease is treated by a different specialist. It doesn't make a lot of sense, but it sure makes a lot of dollars.

The above philosophical lens—creating health via the health model of proper diet, nutrition, adequate sleep, adequate exercise, relationships, stress-mitigation practices— and explanation about healthcare insurance gives you the best perspective through which you can view health and disease. It will be immensely important for reading the rest of this book. Because I can explain the science of autoimmune disease, I can explain the science of why diet and lifestyle can reverse it, and I can show you how to reverse it . . . but if you are still approaching it from the wrong philosophical lens, you will have a difficult time succeeding in getting well.

Chapter 1: What is Autoimmune Disease?

Autoimmune disease, by its most simple definition, is when the immune system, whose normal job is to fight off disease-causing microbes like bacteria and viruses, ends up attacking the body itself. It's a case of friendly fire.

Now depending on what part of the body the immune system attacks, they give the disease a different name. If it attacks your thyroid, it's *Hashimoto's disease*; if it attacks the joints of your hands and feet, it's *rheumatoid arthritis* (RA); and if it attacks your brain it's, *multiple sclerosis* (MS). Now while all of these diseases will present quite differently in terms of symptoms, the mechanism causing them all is essentially the same. That is why they are lumped together as autoimmune disease.

What are the most common symptoms?

While different autoimmune diseases affect different parts of the body depending on where the immune system is attacking, there are common themes as far as symptoms people experience:

Chronic Pain: Pain is somewhere in the body, or all over.

Chronic Fatigue: You always feel tired, no matter how much rest you get or stimulants you take.

Brain Fog: You are unable to think as clearly as you once did.

Digestive Issues: Almost all autoimmune diseases have a digestive component.

Sensitivities: These can vary greatly, but there is usually a sensitivity to at least one thing.

Chronic pain may be in one area, or all over. It could be confined to a specific part of the body like the joints, the muscles, the spine, the gut, or even the reproductive organs. Often it's unexplained, and often it's unresponsive to pain medications.

Chronic fatigue can vary from just a general sense of malaise to crippling fatigue, where working or living a normal life is nearly impossible. But usually there is some lack of energy that neither rest nor stimulants can bridge the gap.

Brain fog may be mild, just having trouble concentrating, or it can be to the point where there is significant cognitive impairment, where it can be difficult to do one's job, be a student in school, or even drive a car.

Digestive issues can vary wildly. It can be as simple as chronic gas and discomfort to chronic constipation, diarrhea, or even blood in the stool. But almost all autoimmune diseases contain a digestive component to them.

Sensitivities can vary. For instance, some people have sensitivities to hot weather and want to move somewhere cold. Conversely, some have sensitivities to cold weather and want to move somewhere warm . . . we have a lot of these where I live, in Arizona. Many are sensitive to certain foods. Smells and chemicals are other ones; in fact, it often goes by its own name, *multiple chemical sensitivity*. These people can have their symptoms flare simply by being around someone with perfume or being exposed to synthetic cleaning solutions. I also see many in the autoimmune crowd who are sensitive to wireless radiation and EMFs (we'll talk more about the health effects of those later).

Another one that I have come across in my years of working with folks with autoimmune disease is sensitivities to emotions. I find that nearly all the people I work with are empathic to some degree. Many often don't realize it, or don't gain this ability until they become sick. They can be sensitive to the emotions of other humans, as well as animals and even plants. This is something I have not seen in the scientific literature, but I have observed empirically just working with autoimmune clients over the years. So if you are reading this and thinking you are the only one, you're not!

Why Do Autoimmune Sufferers Have Sensitivities?

My understanding of this is that for autoimmune folks, their nervous system has been sensitized or over-sensitized. At some point in their life there was trauma(s) that put their nervous system into overdrive. And now in an effort to protect them from future threats, the nervous system is constantly on high alert, and essentially "overreacting" to certain environmental stimuli, whether it be weather, foods, smells, chemicals, emotions, or something else that it perceives as a threat.

Please understand that this trauma is stored in the nervous system and causes it to dysregulate, not just by being overprotective. Understand that fundamentally, the nervous system controls and coordinates all the other systems in the body—including the immune system! So if there is dysfunction in the nervous system, it could potentially lead to dysfunction in any other area of the body—including the immune system!

Later on in this book, I discuss approaches and modalities for clearing the trauma from the body and the nervous system. This process often heals a lot of the sensitivities, as well as helps the body heal from autoimmunity in general.

The Symptoms behind the Symptoms

We've addressed the five most common symptoms of autoimmune disease, but I want to dive deeper. How does that affect us in our everyday lives? After all, autoimmune diseases aren't killing very many people, but they do cause a lot of suffering. And that suffering goes beyond just the physical symptoms. In many ways, those symptoms are just the front-end.

Many people say to me that they feel like their body is in control of them, instead of them being in control of their body. They feel like their body can flare at a moment's notice and plans they made to spend time with friends, to do fun things, or even to complete basic household tasks have to be postponed. Their body and their symptoms run on their own schedule, and they are like a ship in a choppy ocean being thrown around at whim.

As a result, they feel like they can never fully be themselves. They can never fully show up for the things they care about, whether it's with their family, their friends, their partner, their hobbies, their passions, or their work. They are always giving suboptimal effort and are often simply phoning it in.

A main thing people experience is feeling like they have an invisible disease. If you take someone with Crohn's disease, Hashimoto's, MS, or rheumatoid arthritis, oftentimes they won't look like anything is wrong with them on the outside. Maybe if the disease is very progressed, they may display outward symptoms, such as sausage fingers in the case of RA or walking with a cane in the case of MS. But for the most part the disease is invisible. No one can tell you have it just by looking at you. What does that mean? Well, people are less apt to take you seriously that something is actually wrong, such as your friends, family and coworkers, as well as your doctor. If you have no outward signs of being ill, psychologically it's very easy to brush you off as being a hypochondriac or exaggerating just how bad things are. The reality is often the opposite: many people with autoimmune disease are actually pretending that's it's not as bad as it actually is.

So what happens then? No one close to you takes you seriously. It leads to a lot of mental and emotional distress. We feel like people don't understand us. We feel isolated from the people we care about, whom we expect to care about us in return. It's a very lonely, frustrating feeling. Often, we begin to question:

"Am I really this sick?"

"Am I just making this up?"

"What is wrong with me?"

The pain and discomfort we endure daily is multiplied by these feelings of isolation and not feeling understood. Often we retreat into our own little worlds, not wanting to be around people who don't understand. What's worse is that we feel so isolated and so not understood, we think that there can't possibly be a solution. How can there be a solution, cure, or a way out of this if no one else can even *ac-*

knowledge that it's a thing? We grow hopeless thinking that we will be stuck this way forever.

If you're like I was back in 2010, you may think you're the only one. You may think that no one else is having, or has had, this kind of experience. But I want to tell you that you're definitely not alone. There are literally millions of other people suffering with this, and it rarely gets talked about. You're definitely not the only person who is going through this. And you're absolutely not the only person who has friends and family that don't get it and don't understand. The good news is that there is a whole community of people out there who do, you just need to find them. And most importantly, there is hope, there is a way out, and much more often than not, these conditions can be reversed with diet and lifestyle.

A Brief History of Autoimmune Disease

While conditions like rheumatoid arthritis, systemic lupus erythematosus, and multiple sclerosis were discovered in the mid-nineteenth century, the first mention of anything resembling autoimmunity in the scientific literature was in 1904 when scientists first observed white blood cells attacking red blood cells. The term autoimmune disease didn't appear in the scientific literature until about 1940. Up until the late-twentieth century, these diseases were exceedingly rare, and there were far fewer of them. Now there are over two-hundred-plus documented autoimmune conditions.

Now ask yourself, when was the first time you heard the term *autoimmune disease*. Likely you first heard it less than ten years ago. This disease phenomenon has exploded in the past ten to twenty years. In 1997, the first ever estimate of the prevalence of autoimmune disease put it at nine-million Americans afflicted. At the time there were about eighty known autoimmune diseases. Data from 2015 now suggests that the prevalence is twenty-five million diagnosed and twenty-eight million undiagnosed for a total of about fifty-three million Americans affected, with a total of two-hundred known autoimmune diseases. *How in the world did this explosion happen?* We'll explore that in the next chapter

Chapter 2: What is the Cause of Autoimmune Disease?

What Causes Autoimmune Disease?

What causes autoimmune disease? Unfortunately, the answer to that question is up for a lot of debate, and anyone who doesn't give you an extremely nuanced answer is either undereducated on the topic or oversimplifying.

Now the mainstream medical community will generally say one of two things: either (1) "The cause is unknown. We do not know the cause. It just 'happens'" or (2) "Genes cause the disease."

I feel like the first one is the most honest answer they can give. And with mainstream medicine as we'll learn, because of their philosophical approach, they don't really care very much about the actual root cause of any disease. They are so focused on suppression and treatment of symptoms that they usually disregard the root cause for most diseases, especially chronic ones.

This second argument is interesting. Genes cause auto-immune disease. We know that certain genes are correlated with certain autoimmune diseases. These are called HLA (human leukocyte antigen) genes. *Leukocyte* is the technical term for a white blood cell and *antigen* is something that an anti*body* binds to and attacks. So these genes indicate the presence of an antigen on a human cell that the immune system could attack. These genes have names like HLA-B27 and HLA-DR4, which are essentially just the names of genes for different antigens that could appear on cells. Each of these HLA genes is correlated with a different autoimmune disease (or family of autoimmune diseases), because they represent an antigen on a different type of cell in the body.

Now here's where things stop adding up. The gene is *not* an absolute indicator of getting the disease. It is possible to get the disease without having the gene, and it is also very possible to have the gene and never get the disease.

Keep in mind that our genes have been around for literally millions, even billions, of years. But autoimmune disease is a relatively novel phenomenon. Until the twenty-first century, it was so rare, most people, even medical professionals, were not familiar with the phenomenon! In the past twenty to thirty years, the human gene pool has not changed much. Yet the prevalence of these diseases has exploded—now it's believed one in seven American adults have a diagnosed or undiagnosed autoimmune disease! Clearly, the gene pool cannot change that fast.

The likelihood is that genes somehow predispose us to being vulnerable to having an autoimmune disease, but there must be some external factor or factors that ultimately trigger or cause the disease. We will dive into that in more detail. But for now understand that your genes are not your fate, and that there are other factors, most of which are within your control, that can determine your health.

Toxicity as a Cause of Autoimmune Disease

After researching these diseases for over a decade, I'm convinced that the ultimate root cause of these diseases is toxicity. But this raises the question, How does the toxicity cause an autoimmune cascade?

Here's what I believe happens: when faced with toxicity, the body produces exosomes, which we misunderstand as "viruses," in an attempt to expunge the offending toxic agent (or agents), then antibodies attack those exosomes. The exosomes (often mistaken for viruses) look so much like our own tissues that our body gets caught in the crossfire. The immune system attacks the exosomes (our body's attempt to detoxify) *and* ends up attacking our own tissues that appear similar to the exosomes. The autoimmunity is actually a symptom several levels above a deeper, underlying root cause.

We'll delve deeper into how that works later. For now, let's get familiar with toxicity in terms of what it is, where it comes from, how it affects us, and how our bodies heal from it.

Please understand that the body has the ability to detoxify itself and protect itself from toxins, but in the twenty-first-century world, we are so overburdened with toxins from a wide variety of sources that our body cannot keep them all at bay, and the rate they come into our body exceeds the rate at which our body can expunge them. As a result, we carry an ever-increasing backlog of toxicity at all times. Our body is working to try to expunge them, but it is in over its head. Like a canoe with hole that is being bailed out with a bucket, the body is overwhelmed with a task it cannot do fast enough.

In this chapter we'll explore where this toxicity comes from, how the body tries to deal with it, and why ultimately it leads to autoimmunity. Then we'll explore how to actually detoxify the body, what works, what doesn't, and what approaches actually do more harm than good.

Where Does This Toxicity Come From?

There are several places that these toxins come from in our modern world. Here are the most common sources:

- GMO foods and pesticides
- animal foods (meat, dairy, fish, eggs, etc.)
- processed foods
- household products (especially cleaning products)
- pharmaceutical drugs
- vaccines (controversial, yes, I will explain)
- electromagnetic radiation (EMFs) from technology devices

GMO foods and pesticides. Genetically modified foods are a topic of great concern that need to be addressed. I want to preface this by saying that genetic modification is not an inherently good or bad thing. It is a matter of *how* an organism is genetically modified that is of concern.

As GMO proponents will point out, and I agree, that humans have been artificially selecting to breed different plant and animal hybrids for millennia. This is not something I contest. I also want to assert that artificial selection or artificial hybridization is not inherently a good or bad thing. As a corollary, just because artificial selection has yielded good things does not mean that genetic modification has or will yield good things.

My issue is that most genetic modification is done for the sole purpose of getting more pesticides on plants to better protect them from pests. Crops like wheat and soy have been genetically modified to become what's called "Roundup Ready"—meaning that they can be sprayed with large amounts of a pesticide called Roundup and not die. Roundup, whose main ingredient is glyphosate is produced by the Monsanto Company (now owned by Bayer AG), which also invented Roundup Ready GMO wheat, corn, and soy.

Corn has also been genetically modified to produce substantially more of a compound called *BT toxin*. Corn produces this toxin naturally in very small amounts, and it causes insects' stomachs to rupture, killing them. A genetically modified version produces substantially more BT toxin.

Roundup has been implicated as a carcinogen, among many other toxicity claims. In 2015 the World Health Organization declared Roundup a group 2 carcinogen, meaning it was a probable carcinogen. That classification was later rescinded when a substantial shareholder in the Monsanto Company, Bill Gates, donated to the WHO through his non-profit, Bill & Melinda Gates Foundation.

In 2018 and 2019, Monsanto Company lost several civil lawsuits to people who came down with non-Hodgkin lymphoma after continued exposure to Roundup. In one such case, DeWayne Johnson was awarded $39 million for his cancer, and the jury awarded another $250 million in punitive damages because discovery documents showed that Monsanto not only knew about the link with cancer but also deliberately worked to cover it up.

As mentioned previously in this book, accumulated toxicity is a major contributor to autoimmune disease. With Roundup being so toxic and so ubiquitous in most genetically modified foods, eliminating them from your diet is paramount.

Roundup has also been demonstrated to negatively affect the permeability of the small intestine. The small intestine is where we absorb most of our nutrition from our food. This part of us is selectively permeable to nutrients in our food. It absorbs what we need and leaves the rest of our food to travel through the remainder of the intestine, eventually becoming excrement. Roundup damages this inner lining such that it begins to let in things that would not normally be let in, including compounds that are toxic. This damage to the inner lining is called *intestinal permeability*, or more colloquially known as "leaky gut," and is often seen correlated with autoimmunity.

I highly recommend eliminating Roundup Ready GMO foods from your diet. If you are going to eat corn, wheat, or soy (which I don't advise if you are attempting to reverse autoimmune disease), ensure that it is not covered in Roundup. Note that almost all processed foods are made with GMO corn, wheat, or soy. And all conventional animal feed is GMO corn, wheat, and soy. So avoiding processed foods and animal foods is paramount to mitigating exposure to Roundup.

Animal Foods. When we eat animal foods, we are eating the cumulative toxicity of their lifetime (even if it is a shortened one). The animals are exposed to environmental pollutants in factory farm conditions and fed pesticide-laden GMO foods through their entire life. When we eat their bodies, we are absorbing all the accumulated toxicity of their entire lifetime.

This is especially pertinent in fish who live their entire lives in the most polluted part of our planet: our oceans. They have far higher concentrations of industrial pollutants, PCBs, heavy metals, pharmaceutical drugs and anything else that is dumped into our oceans.

To minimize our exposure to toxicity in our food we want to eat as low on the food chain as possible, ideally organic fruits and vegetables that will have the least amount of bioaccumulated toxicity.

Processed Foods. Processed foods are foods that have been chemically and/or mechanically altered in a lab or manufacturing facility. They have been modified by human hands or machines to be far different than what grows out of the ground or off of a tree. They may have been stripped of nutrients in the processing process, but more importantly, they often have had synthetic chemicals added back in.

These synthetic chemicals are completely foreign to our body. If you cannot pronounce it on a food label, it's likely your body has no idea what it is. Your body recognizes it as a threat, and attempts to detoxify it, or add it to the toxic backlog to be dealt with at a later date. This stresses the body to do this and contributes to disease.

The majority of synthetic chemicals additives to food have *not* been tested. Chemicals that are banned in places like the EU are often still allowed in the US. The United States has a term called GRAS (generally recognized as safe), which essentially assumes innocence until proven guilty with food additives. The FDA has essentially said that it does not have the resources to safety test all food additives and neither does the industry, so it will assume additives are safe until research comes out showing that they are in fact harmful. I don't know about you, but that's not something I'm willing to trust. I think it's much wiser to use the precautionary principle and assume foreign synthetic chemicals are *not* safe until we have evidence to demonstrate that they are. You are welcome to believe otherwise, but it will likely be to the detriment of your health.

Household Products. Household cleaning products contain a variety of synthetic chemicals that are toxic to microbes such as bacteria and viruses, and as a consequence, also toxic to us. They may kill bacteria and viruses, but not humans. However, there is a toxic burden they give, which accumulates over time. Exposure here and there may not be enough to cause harm, but on a timeline of repeated exposure or over years and decades, they can begin to cause harm and build up in our system.

Pharmaceutical Drugs. Most pharmaceutical drugs work by suppressing the symptom and not addressing the root cause. They work by actually interfering with the biological processes that produce the symptoms, rather than solving the root cause of the problem. *Symptoms* are biological processes that exist to tell us something is wrong. Addressing symptoms with pharmaceutical drugs is like putting tape on your car's dashboard when the check-engine light comes on. You didn't solve the problem; you just suppressed your body or the car's cry for help.

Interfering with biological processes just to stop symptoms from happening is inherently toxic to the body. For instance, statin drugs attempt to lower your cholesterol. Do they do this by decreasing the amount of cholesterol you eat? No, they do this by interfering with the biological process by which the body naturally produces its own cholesterol. An enzyme in the body that is part of this process called HMG-CoA reductase is inhibited. The drug prevents this enzyme from doing its job. The problem is that this enzyme is not just used in the production of cholesterol but also many other processes in the body. And cholesterol is not just found in artery clots but also is used as a precursor to many naturally occurring steroid hormones in the body, such as testosterone and estrogen. The downstream effects of interfering with this process are numerous including liver and brain problems later in life. So pharmaceutical drugs are another form of accumulated toxicity the body is attempting to expunge.

Vaccines. This is actually one area where we have shockingly clear data that these products can cause autoimmune disease. Traditionally, this is a subject that is highly controversial. I don't take the controversy lightly, and I am happy to provide rock-solid evidence to present my case.

We can say with absolute certainty that vaccines can cause autoimmune disease as a side effect. These drugs are, after all, designed to work directly on our immune systems. Pharmaceutical drugs have side effects, and vaccines are no different. We have both the clinical and epidemiological data to prove this assertion. Let us start with the HPV vaccine Gardasil. The smoking gun for this can be found in the actual package insert for the Gardasil vaccine, which presents the safety data.

As a special resource to keep you updated with the most recent and valid information, the study I'm referencing and the tables and figures of interest there can be found on our book bonus page. Please visit bonus.createhealthbook.com for this study and more reader bonuses.

Now, normally in scientific studies a drug is tested against a placebo. Vaccines are considered a *biologic* and do not need to be tested in a randomized double-blind placebo-controlled study like pharmaceutical drugs do. The testing is much less rigorous than pharmaceuticals, even for drugs like Viagra. The drugs do not even have to be tested against a true, inert saline placebo.

In the case of the Gardasil vaccine, they use three groups. First, the group that receives the vaccine; second, they use a control group that receives a true inert saline placebo (you'll see how this is used to manipulate the data, later). To complicate matters, they use a second control group that is given an injection of what they call AAHS (anhydrous aluminum hydroxyphosphate sulfate). The important ingredient here being aluminum. This substance is also used in the vaccine as an adjuvant. It is a known neurotoxin and is found in the autopsied brains of people who have dementia and autism. Why are they using this as a control group? That is a good question.

First we look at a table for simple adverse events that occur one to five days after getting the shot. Pain, swelling, redness, etc. We show that the vaccine has the highest rates of these minor side effects, while the aluminum adjuvant only has slightly less, and the saline has the least. This is fairly predictable and makes sense.

One thing I want you to notice is the size of the different groups. The Gardasil group is the largest at 5,088, the aluminum adjuvant group is smaller at 3,470 and the saline placebo is less than 10 percent of the size of either of the previous two. Why is this a problem? Well you're about to see how rank scientific fraud is conducted.

Two things jump out at me here. First off, there were a total of 245 people out of 10,706 who contracted an autoimmune disease within six months of getting the Gardasil shot. That is astounding. The rate is 2.3 percent, or about one in forty-four people who got the series of three shots. If that rate of 2.3 percent of a population contracting an autoimmune disease every six months continued because it was "normal," within five years over 20 percent of people would have an autoimmune disease.

Second is that suddenly, there is *only* one control group noted. The aluminum adjuvant only group and the saline placebo group have been *consolidated* into one column. So we can't tell what the rate is for the aluminum adjuvant group versus the saline placebo group. The rates suddenly appear the same. We are being told here that, essentially, the rate is the same for the drug versus the "placebo" and that just in general if people are given a placebo, they have a 2.3 percent chance of spontaneously developing an autoimmune disease over a six-month period.

You do not have to be a genius to see that this constitutes scientific fraud, and extremely poorly orchestrated scientific fraud. You make the saline group so small compared to the aluminum adjuvant group that when you consolidate the data together, all of a sudden, the effect of the aluminum (in the vaccine group or the aluminum adjuvant group) relative to the saline . . . disappears.

What kind of fools do they expect us to be that 2.3 percent of people just spontaneously develop a systemic autoimmune condition within six months of receiving a "placebo"? It's absolute absurdity. If the drug is in fact safe, why can't they show us the number for the saline placebo group individually? Why else would they consolidate? If this isn't gross scientific fraud, and gross negligence by whomever approved this safety study, I don't know what is.

There are of course many other factors that could in theory contribute to autoimmune disease. But, quite obviously, aluminum is the culprit here. Just because we have found one smoking gun doesn't mean that there are others out there. For most vaccines, they are not studied with an inert placebo and the latency period (length of the study) is sometimes only days or weeks, giving us not nearly enough data to really know what is going on. Much more rigorous, further study is needed on this.

EMFs. As the pace of new technology continues to accelerate, one factor that can no longer be ignored is that of electromagnetic fields, or EMFs, that are put off by devices such as mobile phones, computers, cell towers, Wi-Fi, and Bluetooth devices.

Humans are naturally electrical beings. Our nervous system communicates via electrical signals throughout our body (note: the nervous system uses chemical signals as well, and emerging research is showing it also communicates via sound waves too). Wireless signals from cell phones, cell towers, smart meters, Wi-Fi, and other wireless devices can interfere with these electrical signals.

The harm caused by EMFs is one of the most studied phenomena in science. There are over 20,000 published studies over the past century demonstrating harm . . . at levels *below* the FCC guidelines. The FCC is the Federal Communications Commission, which regulates radio, TV, cell phone, and other wireless signals. Unfortunately, the wireless industry has an enormous amount of lobbying power and a stranglehold over the FCC itself, so a lot of these harms do not get talked about.

The actual mechanisms through which EMFs adversely affect your health are numerous, and definitely not fully understood. Explaining the scientific basis for these phenomena goes far beyond the scope of this book.

For the sake of your health, it is important to mitigate your exposure as much as possible. Based on the overwhelming body of evidence, the most common effects of over exposure to wireless are headaches, sleep disturbances, anxiety, heart issues, and brain tumors.

For people with autoimmune disease, and trauma bound up in their nervous system, exposure to EMFs can inhibit the healing process considerably. Most notably, exposure to radiation during night time can interfere with your brain's ability to produce the hormone melatonin. With insufficient melatonin, sleep becomes difficult. Adequate rest is a very important part of healing chronic disease. Turning off your Wi-Fi router at night is probably the single biggest thing you can do to help improve your sleep.

Here is a full list of the best ways to mitigate your exposure:

- Turn your Wi-Fi off at night or when you are not using it. *Especially* if the router is in your bedroom. Due to the inverse-square law, the radiation is exponentially stronger the closer you get to the router.
- Avoid carrying your cell phone on your person when it is on or not in airplane mode. If you must keep it in your pocket, use a faraday wallet, which can block EMFs.
- If you have a smart meter on your home, GET RID OF IT! These give off huge levels of unsafe radiation. Call your power company and tell them you want it removed. They may charge you a fee for this. Try to negotiate that, but it is definitely not worth your health to have one of these.
- If a small cell 5G tower is built near your home, figure out what you can do to either get it moved or have your city write a wireless ordinance to cap the maximum radiation coming off of it. Much more resources are available on this issue at www. scientists4wiredtech.com.

There are many devices out there, such as pendants, stickers, and even water filters, that claim to defend against EMFs. I have not seen demonstrable evidence that any of them work other than faraday wallets, which are essentially a hermetic seal around your device. Mitigating your exposure to the best of your ability by turning them off or staying away from them is your best option.

How Toxicity Likely Causes Autoimmunity

We do know that in autoimmune disease, autoimmune antibodies are present. These are antibodies made by the immune system that attack a specific type or types of cells in the body. For example, in Hashimoto's we can find the presence of anti-thyroid antibodies that attack the actual thyroid.

But this raises the question, *Why* would the body be creating antibodies to attack its own cells? Where has a wire crossed and what has gone wrong such that the body is doing this now? Surely a glitch like this would have a hard time surviving millions of years of evolution.

This always puzzled me, because it did not seem to add up. If the body is this self-organizing, self-healing, self-replicating organism, why would it attack itself? It is a very interesting question that I do not have an entirely clear answer on, but I would like to present you with some ideas that I have come across and some of my own thoughts on the matter.

One of the main theories is that there is presence of a virus in the system that the body is trying to attack. It just so happens that the antigens on this virus are very similar to antigens on human cells. As a result, in an effort to fight off this virus, the body creates antibodies which inadvertently also attack its own cells.

Many clinicians have tested patients with autoimmune disease for various viruses. They find that many are high in certain viruses like Epstein-Barr virus, which traditionally has been associated with a childhood disease called mono-nucleosis. Is this virus somehow still active in the system and the body is trying to fight it, creating antibodies for it that inadvertently cross-react with its own cells? That is one theory.

Now, if we are seekers of truth, the depth of knowledge, and the absolute root cause, it raises the question, Where did these viruses come from? How did some people get in-fected and not others? Are these viruses contagious, and by what means? There is no record of autoimmune disease be-ing communicable by air, touch, sexual contact, or blood-to-blood contact. Whether these viruses are implicated in the cause or not, it does raise the question, Where did they come from?

This is where we begin to question the very idea of the pathogenic model, that viruses always cause disease. In the past twenty years, the explosion in popularity of a phenom-enon called the *microbiome* has burst into the mainstream scientific dialogue. We now know that our body is home to billions of beneficial bacteria that help us with everything from digesting our food to helping us fight infection. This is not to deny the existence of harmful bacteria, they can still cause disease. And good bacteria in the wrong place can also cause disease. For example, E. Coli naturally lives in the large intestine and in the soil. But get that bacteria in your mouth or in your stomach, and you're in for a not-so-pleasant experience.

Similar to the existence of the microbiome, we now know that we have an ecosystem of beneficial viruses called the *virome*. These viruses exist symbiotically within us without causing disease.

We are also beginning to understand that the human body actually creates viruses to use as messengers. Some call these friendly viruses *exosomes*. And these viruses may be created as some way of passing on information about how to combat toxicity and other forms of harm that come at the body.

My theory, as it stands now, for the cause of autoimmune disease is that the primary causative agent is toxicity from a multitude of sources: heavy metals, air pollutants, water pollutants, pesticide residues, artificial ingredients in food, pharmaceuticals, and vaccines, as well as EMFs from: cell towers, cell phones, Bluetooth and Wi-Fi.

The body has detoxification pathways for eliminating these, but as our chronic toxic burden continues to increase as time goes by, eventually the body starts to hit various saturation points where it can no longer remove the toxins at a rate greater than the toxins are coming in. The body begins to accumulate and store the excess toxicity in various organs, most notably the liver, the fascia, and kidneys. As a function of trying to fight the toxicity, the body then begins to produce exosomes, similar to viral particles, but these exosomes have antigens similar to other cells in the body. This is where the autoimmune cascade begins. So ultimately the cascade of cause works like this: The body is over-saturated in toxicity, so the body creates exosomes to expunge toxicity or to act as messengers, which causes the immune system to create antibodies to said exosomes. Then, antibodies cross-react to the body's own cells, resulting in autoimmunity.

So while there is definitely an immune issue, that is not the true root cause. Autoimmunity is only a symptom of the larger scale problem, which is toxicity. So medicine can attempt to modulate, suppress, or otherwise influence the immune system all it wants, but that will never address the root cause. The true root cause is toxicity, and that is what must be addressed in order to truly heal.

Ultimately this is just a theory. What actually happens in the body is still not fully understood. What we *do* know is that when we assist the body in detoxifying itself by providing it the optimum conditions to heal itself, two things happen: (1) acute healing crises and acute detoxification events often happen and (2) the disease remits. So while the intermediary steps between toxicity and symptoms of autoimmune disease may be up for debate, we know that when we detoxify the human organism, it heals itself from autoimmunity (and many other chronic health conditions).

Detoxification Explained

In our modern world we are beleaguered with toxins as I have demonstrated. They are in our air, they are in our water, they are in our food, they are in household cleaning products. We are hit with electromagnetic waves from electronics we use. We are exposed to so many things that even fifty years ago didn't exist. Our brains and bodies still function as if we are apes living in the nonseasonal tropical rainforest. They have no frame of reference for all the things we are now doing to them.

What is miraculous is that our body is extraordinarily good at handling these toxins. The body can store them in the various eliminative organs, most often the liver but also the fascia, the kidneys, the gallbladder and likely other places too. If these toxins stay in our bloodstream, they could cause us significant harm. And if our eliminative organs tried to process them all at once, they'd be overloaded and go into failure.

People normally think of the kidneys as the primary eliminative organ. They filter our blood and send the waste into our urine stream. At the same time, the bowels also eliminate waste. The skin is also a major eliminative organ as so much can be released through our skin and our sweat. When people have acne or other skin eruptions, this is the body's natural detoxification system at work. It is choosing to get rid of toxins through the skin.

The problem now is that we are subject to so much toxicity that our bodies have been tasked to constantly prioritize what to store and what to try to eliminate as we continue to pump ourselves full of toxins from our everyday environment.

Food is probably the source of toxicity that we have the most control over. We can't control air pollution and other environmental factors, except by moving where we live. Food is something we put in our body three-to-seven times per day (or more!) and we have a lot of control over that.

When we begin to eat extremely clean—especially a diet of primarily raw, uncooked, whole organic fruits and vegetables—we significantly reduce our daily toxic load. We reduce it enough that the body gets very excited. Because now instead of having to manage all this incoming toxicity, it can now work on eliminating a backlog of toxicity that has been stored up for months, years, or often multiple decades. This process is called detoxification.

Let us be extremely clear: *the food itself does not detoxify you.* Your body detoxifies itself to the best of its ability at all times. The less the toxic load on it, the more bandwidth it has open to detoxify what it already has stored. The idea that you can take a supplement, a pill, or a food and it will detoxify you is patent absurdity. Your body is already doing that to the best of its ability, and you are either hindering or facilitating the process. The vast majority of people are hindering the process so severely that they will never experience actual detoxification, because their incoming toxic load is far too high. They will just keep adding to their body's toxic backlog until it eventually kills them.

When I first started my journey, I went through some periods of intense detoxification. I can remember my skin breaking out in a painless rash all over my chest and neck for a day and a half and then the rash promptly vanishing. I would

55

have times when I would go to the bathroom and it would smell like alcohol, even though I hadn't drank in months. Or, I went through a few day stretch where it smelled like marijuana even though I'd only tried it a handful of times in my life, and not in many years. This was the process of my body finally purging toxicity that it had stored for decades. I had reduced the incoming toxic load on my system enough that it had the bandwidth to begin releasing these toxins that had been stored in my system all this time.

The body is doing its best at all times. Three-and-a-half-billion years of evolution got us to the humans we are now. The human organism has acquired vast amounts of wisdom evolving over that period of time. This wisdom goes far beyond anything we can learn from in a lab in a matter of a few decades or a few lifetimes. It knows exactly how much toxicity it can handle in the bloodstream; how much it can eliminate through the kidneys, bowels and the skin; and exactly how much needs to get stored. It prioritizes what toxins go where to do it as safely as possible.

I want to caution you against anyone purporting to sell detoxification devices, herbs, or supplements that claim to be able to do the detoxification work for you. The body detoxes best when given optimum conditions to do so. Any detoxification reaction by the body is a response to the stimulus of toxicity. What I mean by this is that any herb or substance that stimulates a detoxification pathway is *inherently toxic*. The idea that you can expose yourself to toxins to better detoxify yourself may sound tempting, but it is ultimately not in your best interest.

This is not a popular opinion in some natural-health circles, especially among some naturopathic and homeopathic doctors. These people subscribe to what I referred to previously as the alternative medical model, not the actual health model. But I have had many people come to me who ended up in the hospital with heart problems or gallstones after using these "herbal detox" formulas. I don't recommend them. I also understand that saying the body detoxifies itself and that you don't need herbal supplements to do so is not good business for these practitioners. I have no interest in selling you magic potions. What I have to share is the knowledge and experience you need to get well, and the motivation and inspiration to follow through and actually implement it.

So yes, your body has the ability to detoxify itself. It is all about providing it with the optimum conditions to do that, and that is what this book will teach you.

CHAPTER 3: APPROACHES FOR TREATING AND HEALING AUTOIMMUNE DISEASE

The purpose of this chapter/section is to educate you on all the different approaches to treating or trying to heal from autoimmune disease. There are many different approaches, philosophies, and treatments. But what I most want to impart to you is to expand your mind around exploring all the different approaches and the fundamental philosophical ideas on which they are based.

It is very easy, especially in today's world, to be caught up in a specific paradigm or set of ideas. When that happens, it becomes very difficult to acknowledge, consider, or check out new information that may challenge that paradigm. But I will tell you, if your paradigm is centered around the idea that mainstream medicine is the only thing that really works, you are likely in for an ever-growing litany of medical conditions along with medications to fight them.

Often, it is ideas we are most resisting that we desperately need exposure to. And without fully understanding an opposing viewpoint, how can we argue against it?

Mainstream Medical Approach

Let me preface this chapter by saying that if the mainstream medical approach for treating autoimmune disease actually worked, I wouldn't have written this book and you probably wouldn't be reading it. But the unfortunate fact is that it not only *doesn't* work, but it is wrought with side effects. The downsides of Western medicine are many, and I will try to summarize them in the most succinct, logical way.

First off, the lens through which modern medicine looks at the human condition presumes many things about the human organism that are simply not true. Modern medicine sees the human organism as inherently flawed and dysfunctional, that your body is destined to get sick, get injured, and fall apart. Modern medicine's job is then to try to fix you, or at the least manage or slow that eventual breakdown. It does not see the body as capable of healing itself. Instead, modern medicine sees itself as the savior to this frail, inherently faulty, and dysfunctional organism. That somehow in just hundreds of years of medical science, we are somehow smarter than the 3.5 billion years of evolution that got us here.

Second, modern medicine rarely concerns itself with the root cause. Instead, medicine focuses on treating and eliminating symptoms. As Thoreau once said, "There are a thousand hacking at the branches of evil to one who is striking at the root."

For example, let's look at high-blood-pressure medications. Now high blood pressure is an interesting topic because it is so ubiquitous and a contributor to the leading cause of death in the Western world: heart disease.

Before we get into how these medications only treat the symptom of high blood pressure, let's get clear on the cause. High blood pressure is caused by a plaquing or clogging of the arteries throughout the body. Heart attacks themselves usually happen when arteries in the actual heart are clogged. Why and how do these arteries clog? Unhealthy, inflammatory foods damage the inner lining of arteries called the *endothelium*. The body attempts to repair this damage by sending clotting factors. If there are high amounts of cholesterol circulating in the blood, that will glob on to these clots, which will eventually turn into plaques. Think of the artery then like a plumbing pipe where a bunch of gunk has built up on the inside. Eventually the pipes do not drain as well. It takes more force to push fluid through a smaller opening. A mostly-clogged drain will take a long time to empty, and a fully clogged drain will never empty. The same goes for your arteries, the more clogged they are, the slower the blood moves through them. As a consequence, the heart must pump harder to get blood to all the tissues in the body at the same rate. This harder pumping results in higher blood pressure. The narrower the aperture, the more pressure is needed to push fluid through it at the same speed.

So how does modern medicine treat high blood pressure? They've gotten incredibly clever at tricking the body into thinking things are OK. These clever tricks you've probably seen advertised on TV that are called pharmaceutical drugs. So let's familiarize you with four of them and how they work.

1) **Anticoagulants.** Commonly known as blood thinners, these interrupt your body's ability to clot its own blood, to try to prevent plaques from being created in your blood vessels. There's just one problem: you kind of need that ability to clot. People on these drugs develop bleeding ulcers that can, in some instances, be deadly. The clotting is a symptom of the body trying to repair itself, and if you interfere with that, you'll have consequences known as side effects.

2) **Diuretics.** These drugs try to lower the volume of blood in the system by dehydrating you so that the heart has an easier time pumping it through narrowed blood vessels. Only problem is, you need that blood. As a consequence, you get dizziness, muscle cramps, and elevated blood sugar. Your body knows how much blood it needs. Bloodletting was a disaster in the middle ages; a higher tech way of doing it is not going to solve the problem.

3) **Beta blockers.** These drugs block something called a beta-receptor, which receives a signal from your nervous system to pump the heart harder. But the only reason the brain wants to pump the heart harder is to overcome all the resistance that has built up in the arteries. When that nervous system signal is blocked, your heart doesn't pump as hard, so you feel weak, dizzy, and tired as a consequence.

The heart pumping too hard is a compensation for a larger problem, not the actual problem itself.

4) **Statins.** These interfere with your body's ability to create its own cholesterol, but do absolutely nothing to stop the cholesterol people are shoving down their face holes three-to-seven meals a day. If the drug slapped the cheeseburger out of your hand, it would be a lot more effective. Your body produces the exact amount of cholesterol it needs, no more, no less. You don't need to shut off that mechanism, and giving it any extra is going to cause problems too. In fact, the enzyme used to make cholesterol that's disabled by statin drugs is used in many other biological processes; as a consequence, these drugs can cause liver damage, brain damage, and diabetes.

What's more, when you're given these drugs, you're told to take them not just for a few weeks or a few months or a year but for the rest of your life. If you take drugs, you're guaranteed to be sick forever, you'll *never* get well. That's the guarantee. Ultimately, we are trying to medicate our way out of problems we have behaved our way into. The numbers speak for themselves: 600,000 deaths a year from heart disease. The strategy isn't working.

This is what happens when we try to treat the symptoms but ignore the root cause. We may prolong life for a little while, but we never solve the problem and often we create other problems in the process that we call "side effects." As I said, if we wanted a drug that treated the root cause of heart disease, we'd make a pill that slaps the cheeseburger out of your hand. Not plaquing your arteries with inflammatory foods but replacing them with healthy, whole plant foods is the way to treat the root cause of heart disease. Anything else is just going to be a waste of time.

Unfortunately, we have the same strategy with autoimmune disease. In attempting to treat the body's symptoms, we ignore the root cause and as a consequence never "cure" the disease, creating a bunch of side effects in the process.

Most notably, biologic drugs continue to skyrocket in popularity as a way to treat autoimmune disease. These are *immune-suppressing* drugs. The thought process is that your immune system is mistakenly attacking you, and therefore the best strategy is to suppress your immune system to stop that from happening. There's just one problem . . . you kind of need your immune system, right? And in 2020 everyone got a very harsh reminder of that.

So what happens when you suppress your immune system? Well, now you're more vulnerable to every cough, cold, skin infection, and bug that comes your way. You've traded in your autoimmune disease for a host of other infectious diseases. With long-term use, many of these drugs list cancer as a side effect. These biologics are the epitome of hubris of the medical system. They literally disable the very system that your body uses to defend against infectious disease, making you that much more dependent on the medical system.

Now the medical system may argue that they are actually treating the root cause of the disease, after all it is the immune system that has gone haywire attacking the body. But if we remember back to the discussion on root cause, the immune system is not actually the root cause of the problem. The root cause of the problem is accumulated toxicity that the body is trying to expunge. Creating virus particles that the immune system attacks is a downstream effect of that, and those virus particles having a similar antigen to some of the body's own cells is a downstream consequence of *that*. So the immune system is actually a tertiary downstream effect, not the root cause itself. After all, it makes zero evolutionary sense that an immune system would start attacking the body for no reason. How would such a trait be naturally selected for on a long timeline? It wouldn't.

Functional Medicine Approach

As frustration and disgust with the traditional medical model grows, people continue to seek out alternatives. One field that has emerged and grown in popularity is that of functional medicine.

Functional medicine differs from traditional medicine in trying to find nonpharmacological ways to work with the body to help it heal. It realizes that pharmaceutical drugs are toxic, and the implications of their side effects on human health can be disastrous.

While functional medicine does urge patients to change their diet, it also focuses on various supplements as well. Many of the supplements are centered around naturally occurring plants and plant extracts that help reduce inflammation in the body. This often gets results that are much better than a pharmacological approach. However, it certainly has its own set of drawbacks and an ugly underbelly.

Functional medicine practitioners get a large percentage of their revenue from supplement sales and are therefore financially incentivized to prescribe supplements to patients (unlike medical doctors who are generally not directly incentivized to sell pharmaceuticals). This means that the more supplements they sell, and the more expensive those supplements are, the more money they make. This incentivizes a behavior where these practitioners begin prescribing laundry lists of supplements, the vast majority of which their patients don't need. And if their patients were able to make the dietary changes I prescribe in this book, they probably wouldn't need almost all of them.

The supplement industry in recent years has become an analog to the pharmaceutical industry. They have put themselves in charge of practitioner education when it comes to chronic disease, whether it be heart disease, diabetes, autoimmune, Lyme disease, or something else. They put on seminars that teach doctors how to diagnose the conditions, as well as treat them, almost invariably with their line of supplements. So doctors come for an education on how to diagnose and treat conditions with functional medicine, and are essentially indoctrinated on how to sell supplements from the company that put on the seminar.

This creates essentially para-pharmacy. Now instead of placing your patient on five pharmaceutical drugs, you are placing them on five (or ten, or fifteen-plus) supplements, with some brief obligatory lip service about diet thrown in. This is the alternative medical model, which, as discussed, is effectively just the medical model dressed in drag.

I've talked to plenty of people who are on a boatload of pharmaceutical medications and not getting any better. I've also talked to dozens of people who are on a boatload of functional medicine supplements and also not getting better. Who is worse off? Does it matter? The important thing is neither group has been educated about a much more effective way that would free them from dependence on drugs and the vast majority of supplements.

This is why although I may occasionally recommend certain supplements like vitamin D3 and vitamin B12, I never sell them, because I do not want a financial incentive to sell something to someone that they don't need. Instead, I base my business around selling education, motivation, inspiration, and accountability that helps people to make the necessary changes in their life to create an amount of health sufficient to reverse disease. Remember: the body heals itself; we are just facilitating that process with our diet and lifestyle.

Low Carb, Paleo, and Keto Diets

This dietary pattern has seen its popularity come and go in waves over the years. Originally in the twentieth century, it was Dr. Atkins who popularized his low-carb diet for weight loss. People were enamored with the idea that it was carbohydrates making them fat, and as a corollary, could eat as much meat, bacon, dairy, and oil as they wanted. Dr. Atkins died in 2003. The autopsy report says that he died from a blow to the head when he slipped on the ice from what appeared to be a heart attack. On the operating table he weighed over 250 pounds, and they found systemic atherosclerosis (plaquing of the arteries) throughout his body. His followers hold on to the delusion that Dr. Atkins was in fact healthy and his brain bleed was simply the result of a bad accident. But his medical records and autopsy report say otherwise.

In the 2000s, Dr. Loren Cordain brought Dr. Atkins failed ideas back with this idea of the Paleo diet. His book asserted that cavemen ate a preagricultural diet of primarily animal foods and vegetables with small amounts of fruit and no grains or legumes. Cordain persuaded people to eat an animal-based diet with some vegetables. It was a rehash of the Atkins diet, but Cordain improved it by telling people to focus on organic whole foods, including plenty of vegetables.

On such a diet, people found that they could see improvement with autoimmune conditions. Removing the processed and GMO foods that caused intestinal permeability yielded some health gains for adopters of this diet. The focus on organic food, whether animal or plant in origin, also contributed to positive health outcomes.

By the late 2000s, its practitioners were beginning to see drawbacks just as the Atkins craze had. On a long enough timeline, people eventually gained their weight back. They noticed other problems, such as body odor, fatigue, reliance on stimulants like coffee, and elevated blood sugar, blood pressure, and blood cholesterol. Eventually the paleo diet was demonized for being unsustainable long-term and riddled with other problems.

Did its followers learn their lesson? Of course not. The low-carb paleo diet re-emerged again as the "Keto" diet sometime around 2013. Apparently low-carb just wasn't low-carb enough, and cutting down to "no-carb" was clearly the solution. Keto devotees slammed the Atkins diets and Paleo diets for allowing too many carbs, for being unsustainable, and even for "not being scientific."

For a diet that supposedly creates health, its loyal followers saw an array of side effects from the initial "keto flu" to the dreaded "keto crotch." Don't worry, a plant-based diet doesn't have side effects, if anything your susceptibility to the flu and strength of body odor will decrease. As a symptom of a lack of fuel to burn, keto dieters often load up on coffee as a stimulant, a very unsustainable strategy for energy. In fact, many low-carb-diet promoters sell their own brand of coffee that they know their followers are desperate for.

Ironically, if going low carb to no carb was the first double down, an offshoot of the movement doubled down again. As if nearly eliminating carbohydrates weren't enough, the "carnivore" diet proclaimed that meat was the only food worth eating and that benefits could be derived from eliminating plant foods altogether. This diet has probably the least amount of evidence to support its use.

The Inuit (colloquially known as the "Eskimo") had lived off a diet that was primarily animal-based before colonization. In low-carb circles these people are celebrated as a population that "thrived" on a meat-based diet. Unfortunately, the scientific record shows that they definitely did not thrive. The average Inuit died at age thirty-nine of osteoporosis. They often had constipation so bad from the lack of fiber in their diet that they would pray to a "fart god" to have a bowel movement. Low-carb bro scientists like to point out that the Inuit almost never died of heart disease or cancer, the top killers of Americans. They want to imply that their meat-heavy diets were somehow protective. But when the average heart disease and cancer deaths happen in your 60s and 70s, Inuits, who die in their 30s and 40s, would never live long enough to die from heart disease or cancer. These are the sort of disingenuous pseudoscientific assertions that the low-carb community have fooled themselves with and are attempting to put their followers under the same deluded spell.

Since these diets demonize processed foods and GMOs while promoting organic, there are some health benefits over the standard Western diet. Many people do report improvement of autoimmune symptoms or even reversal. But with all that, there are still negative long-term health consequences. So while one may be able to reverse autoimmune disease on a low-carb diet, over time they will see weight gain, elevated cholesterol, elevated blood sugar, elevated blood pressure, stimulant dependency, constipation, and a host of other consequences of their actions. Some of these will be life-threatening, some mere inconveniences. A predominantly raw plant-based diet avoids all these negative side effects while still reversing autoimmune disease.

Dr. Ben's Approach: A Plant-Based Diet

The next two chapters will expound on my method and the science supporting it. A plant-based diet of primarily fruits and leafy greens is optimal for human health. All our closest relatives in the animal kingdom (chimpanzees and bonobos) eat a diet of primarily fruits and leafy greens. It is the diet that best meets our nutritional needs, leaves behind the least amount of metabolic waste, and exposes us to the least amount of toxicity.

Chapter 4: The Science of Plant-Based Nutrition

Plant Based Nutrition: Introduction

In order to provide the body-mind with the proper conditions for healing itself, one of the things we must do is feed it the optimum foods. Any foods that are not optimum for the human organism will act as interference against the body-mind's natural self-healing mechanisms.

This of course raises the question: What is the optimum food for human beings? There are a number of ways to try to deduce or induce the answer to this question. I will attempt to derive it from a number of points of view: anthropology, epidemiological data of health outcomes, and clinical data of health outcomes.

From an anthropology perspective, if we want to determine the optimal human diet, we would look at our closest living relatives. Chimpanzees and bonobos share about 98 percent of our DNA, meaning they are the animals on the planet that we are most like. We diverged from a common ancestor about fifteen-million years ago. Given that evolutionary changes can take tens or hundreds of millions of years to develop, there should not be much of a significant difference between our anatomy and physiology.

The chimpanzees eat a diet that is primarily fruit-based. They are a specific type of taxonomy called a *frugivore*, which is different from an omnivore, carnivore, or herbivore. Frugivores eat primarily fruit and tender leafy green vegetables. They have opposable thumbs, which allow for picking of fruit and climbing trees. They have a long digestive tract, about six times their height for digesting plant matter. Their teeth consist of somewhat sharp incisors, with lots of flat molars for grinding plant matter. Frugivores have advanced color vision and are especially good at detecting shades of red, orange, and yellow, which allow us to better detect fruit growing on trees.

From an epidemiological standpoint, we can see that the populations that eat the most whole, unprocessed plant foods and the least amount of animal products and processed foods are the ones with the longest life span—and lowest rates of chronic disease. The China Study, the Epic Oxford study, and the Blue Zones study demonstrate these findings. The Global Burden of Disease study from 2012 shows that worldwide not eating enough fruit is the leading cause of death for all chronic diseases.

Why a Raw Fruit-Based Diet to Reverse Autoimmune Disease?

Much of the literature shows that humans thrive on a plant-based, or mostly-plant-based, diet. According to the study of the Blue Zone regions, i.e. regions with the most centenarians (people living over a hundred years old), locals eat a predominantly plant-based diet. But none of these people eat a 100 percent raw plant-based diet. So why would I advocate for that?

Simply put, a diet of fruits and leafy green vegetables provides the optimum conditions for health. Cooked plants, especially unprocessed ones, can certainly sustain us well. A whole-food plant-based diet can prevent and reverse chronic metabolic diseases, such as heart disease and type 2 diabetes. No other diet than a whole-food plant-based diet can reverse those diseases. They can help us achieve fantastic levels of health.

However, with autoimmunity, the level of toxicity is so high and the lack of health is so dire, we must apply the absolutely optimum conditions for the body to heal itself. One can certainly achieve an improvement in autoimmune symptoms eating a whole-food plant-based diet that includes cooked foods, and in some cases even reverse them. But for most, an entirely raw diet must be sustained for a period of time in order to achieve full reversal. This is the work of creating as much health as possible to overcome a condition that is essentially a very dire deficit of health.

The Downsides of Cooking Food

This section is in no way intended to be raw-food dogma. But there are disadvantages to cooking food that weigh out certain advantages, as we'll talk about. Back before the popularization of the germ theory, eating a lot of raw food was actually a common practice. But when the germ theory became popular, people began to cook their food much more, with the intention of killing germs.

Humans are the only species that cook their food. This provided us with a number of evolutionary benefits for the survival of our species as a whole but was not the best approach for individual health. For example, with grains we could store a food supply that would not go bad for years. So if blight or famine were to occur, we would have a backup food supply. In the absence of other foods, we could find sustenance from meat, provided we cooked it first. It had many ways of keeping us from starving, even if it was never optimal for health.

When you cook food, you derange or destroy many of the nutrients. The carbohydrates become caramelized, a process where chains of sugars bond to each other, making them much harder to digest and actually increasing blood sugar levels when eaten. The heating of carbohydrates also produces a toxic chemical called acrylamide, although in normal amounts of whole plant foods, this is not enough to cause harm.

When protein is cooked, it becomes what we call *denatured*. Long strings of amino acids comprise proteins, but these amino-acid strings now tangle and bond on to each other in random places, making them much harder to break down, digest, and assimilate. For example, if you took hair, which is made out of a protein called keratin, and you put it near a flame, then tangled it, the hair would actually bond to itself becoming a tangled mess you could not undo. The same thing happens with any protein you expose to heat. As such, most cooked protein the body is unable to fully digest or use. Excess may even produce an inflammatory effect in the body, giving the appearance of bigger muscles, but oftentimes these muscles are just marbled with excess inflammation.

Fat is probably the worst of the macronutrients to expose to heat. When it heats, it oxidizes and becomes carcinogenic (causes cancer). At very high temperatures, the cis bonds actually turn to trans bonds, creating what are called trans fats. These fats have no nutritional value to the human organism and are actually carcinogenic.

Raw food on the other hand has maximum nutrition because it is in its whole, natural state. It will digest the best and be easily broken down for energy. Raw fruits and vegetables also have the least amount of toxicity. Without the toxic load of cooked foods, processed foods, and animal foods, the body can begin to clear the backlog of toxicity it has accumulated in the various parts of the body: the liver, the skin, the connective tissue, the lymphatic system, and so on. This is why raw foods are so powerful at helping you detox. They have no inherent detoxification ability themselves, but since they present such a minimal toxic load, they free up the body's natural detoxification pathways.

Also, since the body needs to use minimal energy to digest and assimilate these foods, vital energy from the body is freed up for healing. This freeing up of vital energy is what allows us to reverse autoimmune disease on a raw fruit-based diet.

The B.I.G. Fallacy

One of the most common pitfalls I see people make in nutrition is to look at foods through a *reductionist* lens. They want to look at individual components of the food that are considered healthful and then ignore other components of the food that are unhealthful. This is a foolish way to approach nutrition, because if we don't look at the big picture of how a food affects us overall, we are going to miss the forest for the trees.

People will come up with all kinds of rationalizations and justifications for the unhealthy foods that they eat, simply because they contain one or two nutrients that they are told they need. I call this the B.I.G. Fallacy, the "But It's Got" fallacy:

"You mean milk is unhealthy? But it's got calcium!"

"You mean meat is unhealthy? But it's got protein!"

"You mean beer is unhealthy? But it's got vitamin B6!"

"You mean cocaine is unhealthy? But it's got antioxidants!"

And you can see where this eventually leads. Almost any food can be justified as healthy if we only look at the nutrients it does contain and ignore all the unhealthy things that come along with it.

We have to look at the big picture. We have to choose foods that best meet our nutrient needs. We have to choose foods that contain what is healthful and that don't contain what is not healthful. Anything less, and we are kidding ourselves that it's healthy; otherwise we are falling for the B.I.G. Fallacy.

Macronutrients: Carbohydrates, Protein, and Fat

My intention here is to clear up a lot of the misunderstandings, and overgeneralizations, about these various macronutrients. I want to expound on each one and their role in nutrition and your health. A lot of this will be explained in a completely different context than what you may have learned, so keep an open mind and prepare to have your paradigm challenged.

What's most important to understand is that no single food can be defined simply by its majority macronutrient content. That is, the idea that some foods are "carbs" or "protein" or "fats" is a gross overgeneralization of the science that leads to misunderstandings and misapplication of the science. All foods contain all three to varying proportions. The only way to remove one or more of these macronutrients is to *refine* the food, which by definition removes nutrition from it. That is, the only "foods" that are pure carbohydrates are sugar in powder form. The only "food" that is pure protein is protein powder (and that is difficult to get to be 100 percent only protein), and the only "food" that is pure fat is oil. Sorry to burst your bubble but— these refined foods have had nutrition removed from them, they can no longer be considered health foods.

Plant-Based Nutrition: Carbohydrates

To understand carbohydrates, we need to break them down into two subsets. Most often, people look at the two types of carbohydrates as *simple* and *complex*. A simple carbohydrate is a sugar like glucose, fructose, or sucrose. A complex carbohydrate would be a chain of these carbohydrates forming a longer molecule. While there are definite differences in these, and how they are metabolized, there is a far more important distinction that needs to be made.

What most people fail to look at is the idea of *whole* versus *refined*. They paint carbohydrates with a wide brush. They see donuts and mountain dew as equivalent to sweet potatoes and mangos. Thankfully, it doesn't work that way.

Donuts and soda are *highly* refined foods. Neither of them grow out of the ground. They go through multiple chemical- and mechanical-separation processes to get to the end product. During these refining processes, almost all constituent nutrients are removed from the original plants these were made from. For instance, in high-fructose corn syrup the fat and sugar are separated out to make corn syrup and corn oil.

In this process, the fiber, the vitamins, the minerals, the protein, the antioxidants, and the phytonutrients are removed. And so you are left with pure sugar (corn syrup) and pure fat (corn oil), with no other nutrition in them. These are not health foods.

Donuts on the other hand do not even have most of their calories coming from carbohydrates. They are deep-fried in oil, which is extremely calorically dense, causing most donuts to have over 60 percent of calories from fat.

Mangos and sweet potatoes, on the other hand, grow out of the ground. They are a complete nutritional package with vitamins A, B, C, E, and K, minerals, fiber, phytonutrients, enzymes and coenzymes. When eaten in their whole state, they promote health and enable the body to reverse and resist disease.

Carbohydrates in whole plant foods do not raise blood sugar. It's a common misunderstanding that carbohydrates increase blood sugar. Refined carbohydrates certainly can, but carbohydrates coming from whole plant foods do not. How is this so?

Whole plant foods are rich in fiber, which has three main roles in the body: ensuring bowel motility, feeding beneficial bacteria, and helping regulate blood sugar. The fiber actually slows down the uptake of sugar from the digestive tract into the bloodstream. So when you eat a piece of fruit in its whole form or in a smoothie with the fiber intact, the sugar in it has its absorption slowed down by the fiber, so the blood sugar doesn't spike.

If you think about anyone you know with type 2 diabetes, they didn't get it eating mangos and pineapple. They got it eating a standard American diet of junk food. The good news is that a whole food plant-based diet high in whole plant carbohydrates and fiber can actually reverse type 2 diabetes.

A note about low-carb diets. So in the ten-plus-years of doing this, I have seen many trends come and go. Low-carb diets fade in and out of style in cycles so much it's comical. First it was Atkins (then he died of a heart attack), then it was Paleo and Primal, which fell out of favor for not being low-carb enough. Along came Keto, which has been a trend for a few years, but even Keto was thrown under the bus for not being restrictive enough as meat-only carnivore diets have been popularized.

What is unfortunate is that in all these low-carb or no-carb diets, the "carbs" that are always demonized are refined junk foods with most of the nutrition removed. Bread, donuts, pizza, and cinnamon rolls are rightly blamed for weight gain. But then fruit and other whole plant foods that are predominantly carbohydrates are thrown under the bus with them. It's a false equivalency. But this is what happens when we have a reductionist view of the science. Studies on high-fructose corn syrup's pathogenic effects on the body are shown, and the fructose in fruit is demonized as equivalent. But refined fructose in high fructose corn syrup with no fiber or other constituent nutrients behaves completely differently than the fructose in a pineapple with the fiber intact. This painting of carbohydrates with a broad stroke has caused low-carb dieters to miss out on a plethora of health-promoting whole plant foods. This is a topic that could turn into an entire book, but I will leave it at this for now.

Plant-Based Nutrition: Protein

This seems to be a vastly contested topic that never really goes away. Perhaps it's due to the fact that the term "protein" comes from the Latin words meaning "of prime importance". Proteins are the building block of so many structures in our bodies it would be easy to think that consuming large amounts of protein is best for optimal health. In this chapter we'll explore why that might not actually be the case, why the type of protein is very important and how much really is optimal.

Where does protein come from? First off, since this seems to be the most common thing to overlook, is that all plants contain protein. Just as protein is a key component of so many structures in humans, so it is in plants. In fact, all animals get protein from eating plants at some point in the food chain, even if they are carnivores. Animals *cannot* create all the amino acids on their own, other than recycling what they already have. This idea that cows, pigs, and chickens are a "sources of protein that we cannot get anywhere else" is quite foolish. Why would those animals be able to get an abundance of protein from the plants that they eat, or somehow transmute the plants that they eat (that supposedly have no protein) into protein? And yet humans cannot do this? There are many places that logic falls apart. Either there is protein in plants, and humans and other animals can get protein by eating those plants, *or* if there isn't protein in plants (spoiler alert: there is plenty), then animals—including humans—should be able to manufacture the needed protein on their own. It turns out it's definitely the former scenario, and we'll go into depth on that next.

Protein Content of Common Foods

Bananas	4%	Strawberries	7%	Cucumbers	11%	Broccoli	20%
Grapes	4%	Watermelon	7%	Tomatoes	12%	Lettuce	22%
Mangos	5%	Potatoes	7%	Apricots	14%	Cheddar Cheese	26%
Cherries	6%	Peaches	8%	Spaghetti	14%	Asparagus	27%
Carrots	6%	Ice Cream	8%	Cabbage	15%	Spinach	30%
Oranges	7%	Rice	8%	Kale	16%	Beef	50%

How much do humans need? If you ask most people why consuming large amounts of protein is important, they will often tell you three things: they need it for energy, they need it to be strong, they need it to be healthy. We'll explore why all three of these things are not, in fact, true.

Human protein needs have been vastly overstated by many authorities, such as the USDA (United States Department of Agriculture) and the AND (Academy of Nutrition and Dietetics). The human body, which in adulthood generally just maintains the same weight, has the ability to recycle its own protein, putting human protein needs only around 2.5–5 percent of calories. But modern nutrition guidelines have put in a margin of safety, doubling the requirement to 10 percent. Eating whole plant foods will generally put a person around 7–10 percent of calories from protein, whereas a person on a Standard Western Diet gets about 16 percent. People seeking to add muscle mass will consume more calories, but do not need to consume a higher percentage of those calories from protein.

Our body breaks down protein into amino acids to use itself. Proteins are long strings of amino acids. The body has to break them down into constituent amino acids and then use those to build its own proteins. When we cook foods, we denature the protein, where in these complex structures, amino-acid strings mush together, fold in on themselves, and become a tangled mess that is difficult for the body to break down. As a result, it is harder for the body to extract all the amino acids out of such proteins. So while animal foods may be higher in overall protein, the body's ability to absorb the actual amino acids in them is inhibited.

Normally protein quality is measured based on a person's ability to add on mass. Protein quality is not measured upon their overall health outcomes. One can easily add mass and strength on a plant-based diet, as long as adequate calories are being consumed. Animal protein is actually high in elements that have a net inflammatory effect on the body: phosphorus, chlorine, and sulfur. Many bodybuilders you see have muscle mass that is marbled due to high amounts of inflammation, which adds to their size but detracts from their health.

What about protein deficiency? Pop quiz: What are the names of the diseases caused by not eating enough protein? Answer: there is only one, and it only happens in cases of starvation. People are so paranoid of "not getting enough" protein, yet many of the major killers in Western society are due to heart disease, cancer, diabetes, and so on, which are all from an excess of too much animal protein.

Protein deficiency only occurs in third-world countries where people are starving. The condition is called *kwashiorkor*, and is essentially never seen in the developed world. Yet many people are consciously trying to consume excess protein in the form of animal products, powdered supplements, drinks, and other products to "get their protein," something they definitely do not need to consume in excess.

The complete-protein myth. Another common myth about protein is that vegetarians cannot get "complete protein"; therefore, they must constantly combine foods to get enough. The creator of this theory, Frances Lapp Moore recanted this idea on his death bed. The fact is that all plants have a complete amino-acid profile. There is no need to specifically work to combine plant foods for a "complete" protein. Simply eating adequate calories of any whole plant foods will provide sufficient (and not excess) protein.

Whey protein is an industrial-waste by-product. The ever popular whey protein is a by-product of the dairy industry. When cheese is made, the whey is separated from the curds. Whey is considered so damaging to the environment that the EPA does not allow it to be dumped on the land. But, the FDA considers it a safe product for human consumption. So the whey is dehydrated and turned into powder, then sold as a health product because of its high-protein content. This is a substance that is too toxic to dump on the land, yet somehow safe for human consumption. Welcome to America where you can take industrial waste, market it with some flashy pictures of fit people flexing, sell it at a huge markup, and make a fortune poisoning people.

What's the alternative to whey protein? I do not recommend taking any protein supplement. As stated, most people in the developed world consume too much protein. Protein powder, even if it's made from a plant source like hemp, rice, or peas, is still heavily refined, with most of the nutrition gone. You are far better off just eating hemp seeds, rice, or peas than taking in a refined powder with most of the other nutrition removed. Bottom line: get your nutrition from whole plants, not powders in a can.

Denatured protein. Protein is formed by chains of amino acids. Any protein that the body consumes, it breaks it down into these constituent amino acids, then uses them to form its own proteins. So this idea that you can grow muscle simply by eating the muscle of a cow, chicken, or pig is nonsense. Your body breaks that tissue down, and the protein found inside into amino acids, then builds its own proteins from that. The idea that you can eat animal flesh and gain its strength is rather shortsighted and sophomoric.

For instance, in some indigenous cultures it is believed that a tiger is a symbol of virility. These people believe that if men have erectile dysfunction, it can be cured by eating the dried penis of a tiger. That somehow the sexual virility and

87

ferocity of this animal will be acquired by you if you eat its sexual organ. To anyone in the modern Western world, this sounds absolutely absurd that you could acquire an animal's perceived sexual prowess simply by eating its sexual organs. Yet, somehow we are willing to accept a similar absurdity, that by eating the muscle of another animal, we are able to acquire its physical strength. Both ideas are utter nonsense.

Plant proteins are generally shorter chains than animal proteins and are easier for the body to break down. The more complex the protein is in terms of length of amino acid sequence and overall structure, the more difficult it is for the body to break down. By cooking, especially animal protein, we do something denature it; wherein, the amino acid chains become jumbled and tangled like a matted part of a dog's fur. These proteins are incredibly difficult to break down, and most of them will leave the body as waste to be processed by the kidneys.

Excess protein is toxic. Consuming more protein than needed, especially from animal sources, is toxic. The human body cannot use, store, or absorb this excess protein. It ends up going to the kidneys, which need to do work to excrete it. This taxes the kidneys and can over time inhibit their ability to do their job.

It is hard to point to one particular aspect of meat and animal protein and to say *that* is the part that specifically causes disease. The saturated fat, cholesterol, TMAO (Trimethylamine-oxide), and excess protein all play a role. Many of the famous bodybuilders of yesterday have had to have multiple heart surgeries and bypasses due to all the animal products they consumed during their careers.

And yet, now we see many plant-based bodybuilders and strength athletes competing and winning in competitions with omnivores.

Plant-Based Nutrition: Fat

Fat can be a very confusing topic, because unlike carbohydrates or protein, it is much more complex and nuanced. There are many different kinds of fat. Some of them "good" and some of them "bad," but even the "good" ones should be consumed in a somewhat limited fashion. This is a complex, nuanced topic, and I have broken down the different types of fat out there, delineating what is to be avoided and why and what I recommend you consume and in what amounts.

Whole-food fat vs. refined oils. One of the most important distinctions we can make is the difference between fat in whole-food form, packaged with its constituent nutrients, and refined fat, which presents usually in a liquid state. I only recommend getting fat from whole plants, not from refined sources.

To demonstrate this idea, let us imagine we are making olive oil. We take olives and we press them in an industrial machine that squeezes out the oil. What is left behind of the olive? Well, pretty much everything but the fat. Left in the press is the fiber, the water, the protein, the carbohydrates, the vitamins (a little bit of fat-soluble vitamin E stays in the oil), the minerals, the phytonutrients, and the enzymes. Wow, we just left behind a lot of nutrients!

Furthermore, the nutrient that we did manage to salvage—the fat—is now set to spoil and rancidify as soon as it is stripped of the fiber and exposed to air. Pure fat with no vitamins, minerals, or fiber is a refined food, just as pure sugar with no vitamins, minerals, or fiber is a refined food. They are both empty calories. And wow, what empty calories oil is! Just one tablespoon is 120 calories of pure fat, with no vitamins or minerals in it.

There seems to be some sort of pervasive myth that the certain types of oil are better than others. That somehow olive oil or coconut oil is good oil but other sources are bad oil. It's like trying to argue that brown sugar is healthier than white sugar or corn syrup. It's all nutritionally replete, empty-calorie junk! Don't kid yourselves. Eat olives, eat coconuts, eat avocados, and the original plants from which these oils are extracted. But eating the junk-food, refined versions of them is not going to serve your health!

The different types of fat: omega-3 vs. omega-6. In terms of how much they can affect your health, omega-3 and omega-6 fatty acids are of prime importance. As a general rule, omega-3's are anti-inflammatory and omega-6's are pro-inflammatory. Since both types of fats are processed by *desaturase* and *elongase* enzymes in the body, the ratio you eat of these two types of fats is extremely important. If you are consuming an excess of omega-6 fats, they will hoard your desaturase and elongase enzymes; your body won't be able to metabolize as much omega-3, which is vitally important. The body doesn't actually need much omega-3 or omega-6, *but* if omega-6 is in gross excess (like it is for most Americans on the standard American diet), the body won't be able to process and use the omega-3's it's getting, even if it's getting more than most others. The optimal omega-3:omega-6 ratio is somewhere between 1:1 and 1:2. If you are consuming more than double the amount of omega-6 than you are omega-3, your body will not likely be able to metabolize sufficient omega-3. Most Americans are consuming around 1:10 or even 1:20.

Omega-6 fatty acids are generally found in processed cooking oil like canola oil, rapeseed oil, soybean oil, and the like. Any fried food is going to be loaded with omega-6 (as well as trans-fat, which we already mentioned). Fried foods, especially fried animal products, are some of the most health-destroying foods a human can eat.

Omega-3 fatty acids are found in fruits and vegetables, but generally in small enough doses that they alone cannot provide sufficient amounts. I recommend consuming omega-3 rich raw seeds, such as chia, hemp, or flax seeds on a regular basis.

I do *not* recommend consuming any of these in their nutritionally devoid oil forms, such as flax seed oil or hemp seed oil. These extracted oils, like all oils, begin to rancidify as soon as they are exposed to air. They are nutritionally bankrupt already, stripped of so many other constituent nutrients, but add on to the fact that the omega-3 oils they purport to provide are already rancidifying before you've picked it off the store shelf.

Fish and fish oil have also been a popular source of omega-3s. Please understand that fish themselves do not create omega-3s, they get them from eating algae that's in the sea. I am also not a fan of eating algae or seaweed. As you may or may not be aware, the oceans are heavily polluted with toxic metals like mercury and aluminum, PCBs, and pretty much every industrial waste product and pharmaceutical drug known to man. So when you are consuming fish, fish oil, or seaweed products, you are getting a toxic package of pollutants along with it. Do not fall victim to the B.I.G. Fallacy ("but it's got omega 3s!"). There are safer, more nutritionally complete ways to get omega-3 fatty acid, without the horrific toxin load.

Fish oil is *not* needed for EPA and DHA. Some animal food proponents, especially those selling fish-oil supplements, will state that it is difficult to convert ALA (an essential omega-3 fatty acid) into the forms that the body most readily uses: EPA and DHA.

This is true in some conditions, but not in others. Allow me to explain. You will have difficulty converting ALA to DHA and EPA if you are consuming a large amount of omega-6 fatty acids from fried and processed foods. The omega-6 pathway will hog the same desaturase and elongase enzymes that the omega-3 pathway likes to use; thereby inhibiting the body's ability to convert ALA into DHA and EPA.

Conversely, if you eat a good ratio of omega-6 to omega-3, preferably 2:1 or 1:1, converting ALA to EPA and DHA should be no problem. Therefore, the ratio of omega-6 to omega-3 is actually more important than how much omega-3 you are consuming. Since omega-6s are so inflammatory, there is only so much the omega-3s can do if you're stifling them by consuming too much omega-6.

Trans-fat. When fats, especially oils, are heated at high temperature, their cis bonds can flip and become trans bonds. These fats are called *trans fats*, and they are not found in nature. They can only be created through high heat. As such, they are completely nutritionally worthless, and as a matter of fact, are carcinogenic! This is another reason fried food is so unhealthy.

Saturated fat, unsaturated fat, and cholesterol. Unsaturated fat, categorized as mono-unsaturated fat (MUFA), and poly-unsaturated fat (PUFA) are generally found in much more abundance in plants than animals. While some plant foods do contain saturated fat, it is much rarer in the plant kingdom. Animal fats are typically 80-percent saturated and 20-percent unsaturated, while plant foods are 20-percent saturated and 80-percent unsaturated.

Saturated fats mean they have no carbon double bonds, only single bonds (i.e., that all carbons are "saturated" with hydrogens). Chemically this makes them very difficult for the body to break down or use.

The primary thing that the body uses saturated fat for is to create cholesterol, which is used as a substrate to create a class of hormones in the body called *steroid hormones*. Steroid hormones include testosterone, estrogen, progesterone, and vitamin D.

While this may be a good thing, an excess of saturated fat and an excess of cholesterol in the system will lead to atherosclerosis, which is the hardening of the arteries, leading to high blood pressure and heart disease.

Most people on the standard Western diet consume far too much saturated fat from animal products and put themselves at risk for heart disease. The body can get all the saturated fat it needs from plants, and excess is harmful. Furthermore, cholesterol is not an essential nutrient. Plants have effectively no cholesterol, yet the body can synthesize what it needs from the saturated fat it does get. As usual, the goldilocks principle applies and an excess of saturated fat is harmful.

Vitamin B12

This always seems to be a controversial subject. B12 is not found in plant foods; it's not made by plants. It's true. You will almost invariably need to supplement. What most people don't seem to understand is that it's not made by animals either. It's made by bacteria. These bacteria most commonly live in your large intestine and in the soil. As humans, we used to be exposed to much more B12 when we grew our own food and when we often ate our food without washing it. But now in our very clean, antiseptic world, we come into contact with dirt and microbes a lot less frequently. It's not just a problem for humans, it's a problem for animals too. So commercial livestock are injected with B12, which is why it can be found in animal products. So if you are getting B12 from eating animals, you're supplementing too, just indirectly.

The B12 that is produced in our large intestine comes out in our excrement and would in theory go back into the soil if it weren't for modern day plumbing. The B12 that is produced by bacteria in our large bowel happens too far down the process for us to reabsorb that B12. But I want you to be aware that it is being produced there. This leaves our options for getting B12 to

1) eating dirt,
2) eating excrement,
3) eating animals, who have been supplementing, and
4) taking a supplement ourselves.

My preference would be number four. Personally, I supplement with an injection once a quarter from my doctor and get on with my life. I recommend this approach, although you want to make sure that the B12 supplement you are taking is high quality and does not have any toxic preservatives or excipients. Most notably, some injectable brands have aluminum, which is extremely neurotoxic and to be avoided. Since some people have an issue producing something called *intrinsic factor*, which helps absorb B12 in the gut, I recommend getting an injection over taking an oral supplement. Since many people, especially those with autoimmunity, can have the MTHFR gene, I recommend a methylated form of B12. So the ideal scenario is getting an injection of methylcobalamin (instead of cyanocobalamin or hydroxocobalamin), which does not have any toxic preservatives or excipients.

Phytonutrients

While science has been able to discover, isolate, categorize, and study many vitamins and minerals, there is a class of nutrients that is still an uncharted frontier in nutrition. That is the class of nutrients called *phytonutrients*, which literally means "plant nutrients." You have probably heard of more well-known ones such as *lycopene* and *resveratrol*. While we have discovered many, scientists estimate that there are thousands of these phytonutrients in plants that they have yet to discover.

These nutrients can really only be found in plants in their whole, natural state. As soon as you subject plants to heat, chemical processing, and so on., these fragile nutrients are often destroyed. As such, no supplement, powder, pill, or potion can really fully substitute whole, fresh ripe, raw, organic plants.

There are so many misconceptions around some phytonutrients such as lycopene, found in red fruits like tomato and watermelon, that suggest if you cook it you make it more bioavailable. This is in some sense true, but you destroy so much lycopene in the cooking process that you would actually absorb more lycopene by not cooking your tomato and consuming considerably more lycopene that just didn't happen to be bioavailable.

Alcohol and Resveratrol. Resveratrol is another phytonutrient that is touted for its prevalence in grapes, especially in wine. This idea that somehow consuming a toxin such as alcohol, which kills any life it comes into contact with, can somehow be made healthy by the fact that it has resveratrol is a concept that makes a lot of dollars, but it does not make a lot of sense. This is the classic application of the "But It's Got" B.I.G. Fallacy: that somehow some boutique phytonutrients cancel out the fact that you are consuming a toxin, albeit in small doses.

Those of us who are experiencing optimal health will feel the negative effects of alcohol immediately upon drinking it, with hangover symptoms such as headache, fatigue, and sinus pain. Those with a tolerance who have been consuming it for a long time will likely notice nothing, as their body is used to experiencing less than optimal health.

Wine and other forms of alcohol are essentially fermented plants, plants that have undergone a controlled spoil in set conditions. If you were eating a bowl of grapes, and one of the grapes was fermented, when you put it in your mouth you would immediately notice and likely spit it out. But when this process is done on a mass scale, the fermented liquid goes through a refining process and is then bottled in a fancy bottle, sold at large markup suddenly, and what was once a clearly unhealthy, spoiled food substance becomes a supposed health-promoting liquid. I hope you aren't fooled.

The Importance of the Microbiome and Virome

In the last fifteen years, the emergence of the topic of the microbiome has exploded into the mainstream discussion around health, wellness, and science. The microbiome is the concept that humans exist symbiotically with a host of different beneficial bacteria throughout our body. These bacteria are so numerous (about 100 trillion) they actually outnumber human cells (15 trillion) in quantity but are only a small fraction of our total mass. These bacteria help us with a number of functions, from digesting food to fighting off infectious disease. We have evolved with them over time and cannot live without them. While they are technically not "us," their symbiotic relationship with us is woven into our very biology and evolution. The average human intestine has over five hundred different species of bacteria.

Different bacteria populate different parts of our body. Often times these bacteria are beneficial to us where they naturally reside but can cause problems if they are transported to other areas of the body. For example, *Staphylococcus aureus* is naturally occurring on the surface of our skin. But if this bacteria gets in our blood, or worse yet travels to our bones, it can cause serious infections, known as a staph infection. The E. coli bacterium is normally found in our large intestine, and in the soil as well. But get that bacterium in your mouth or in your stomach, you are in for a very unpleasant case of food poisoning. If the bacteria from our large intestine accidentally migrate to our small intestine, it can cause a very unpleasant condition called SIBO, or small intestine bacterial overgrowth. These bacteria have very specific homes in certain parts of our bodies, and migrating elsewhere can actually be very harmful for us.

What's fascinating, and applicable here, is that a vast spectrum of different bacteria live in various parts of our gut. These bacteria are symbiotic with us and actually eat our food along with us. As mentioned, the good ones will actually help us break food down. While fiber is an essential nutrient for humans, we can't actually break it down ourselves. It still provides many benefits to us in its unaltered state. But good bacteria in our gut can actually break down fiber and digest it. So one of the three main benefits of fiber is that it feeds good gut bacteria; this property of fiber is why it's called a *prebiotic*.

What's also fascinating is that healthy foods like whole plants will feed the beneficial bacteria, while animal products and processed foods will feed their own cadre of unhealthy bacteria. These bacteria have evolved to become extremely intelligent. When the bad bacteria die off from people eating too much health food (gasp!), they will attempt to preserve themselves by tricking the body into craving the food they like. These bacteria can actually produce neurotransmitters for cravings and send them retrograde up the *vagus nerve*, which goes directly to and from the gut to the brain. Personally, I find this information fascinating, that these bacteria can have such an influence on our behavior, causing us to crave the unhealthy foods that keep the unhealthy bacteria alive.

Should I take probiotics? It would seem that the logical answer to restoring proper gut microbiome balance would be to take a supplement of bacteria called *probiotics*. But if you are not feeding your body the right foods, this is akin to trying to sow seeds for kale on the beach. You can put them down, but if the fertile environment isn't there for them to grow, nothing will happen.

Furthermore, many studies have shown that probiotic supplements are not reliable. For instance, a 2008 study looked at fourteen common brands, and researchers found that only one contained the actual species that were on the label. Furthermore, many had bacteria inside that were already dead and didn't grow.

Should I eat fermented foods? Another approach to getting probiotic bacteria is to consume fermented foods that contain high amounts of bacteria. Fermented foods have basically gone through a controlled spoil and, therefore, have a lot of beneficial bacteria.

Note that once again, if you are eating unhealthy foods along with some fermented foods, the benefits will be minimal. Fresh fruits and vegetables are still the best. But if you are going to eat fermented foods, you want them to be fermented plants like sauerkraut or kimchi, not fermented animal foods as I'll explain.

A hot trend is dairy products advertising themselves as healthful because they have beneficial bacteria. This is another incidence of the B.I.G. Fallacy rearing its ugly head. Just because cow-milk or goat-milk yogurt has probiotics in it, it doesn't dismiss the lactose, cholesterol, TMAO, steroid hormones, saturated fat, and absence of fiber in it. The presence of one good thing can never outweigh the presence of a slew of bad things. Real health foods have all benefits and no side effects.

In addition to a beneficial microbiome of symbiotic bacteria, emerging research is showing that we also have a similar symbiotic relationship with beneficial viruses. These viruses live symbiotically with us and do not cause disease. It's theorized that these viruses act as messengers either within our bodies or from person to person, a way of sharing data and genetic information. This is a topic I have just begun to dive into myself and believe there could be a tie-in with autoimmunity. I hope to share more of what I learn in future books.

Chapter 5: How to Eat to Reverse Autoimmune Disease

Now that I have explained the fundamentals of plant-based nutrition and established that fruits and vegetables are the healthiest foods for humans, let's dive into real-world application. How do you eat a diet of primarily fruits and leafy greens in the real world? Obviously, carrying around a bag of fruits and vegetables with you everywhere you go will work, but it won't be practical. Having eaten this way for over a decade myself, I wanted to lay out a practical primer that anyone could use to get started. How do we go about, in a practical way, eating a diet that is primarily fruits and leafy green vegetables?

1. The primary staple must be fruit. Vegetables, as health promoting as they are, from a caloric standpoint cannot be the primary source of calories. A head of lettuce has 100 calories. One would need to eat twenty to thirty heads of lettuce in a day to sustain their caloric needs.

2. Leafy greens are important, I suggest eating one to two heads of them a day. While they will make a great deal of the diet in terms of volume, the vast majority of the calories will come from fruit.

3. Fruit is seasonal, so the type of fruit will vary with the time of year. At present time of writing this, it's January 2021, and for breakfast I am drinking a smoothie made of one liter of fresh orange juice (that I squeezed myself) with two small papayas blended into it. Right now citrus, papaya, bananas, and persimmons are my staples. In April, mangos, mulberries, and stone fruit will come into season. Then in the summer, berries and melons will come along. In the fall, it will be dates, apples, pears, and grapes. Those are of course just a fraction of the varieties of fruit that are available throughout the year.

4. Bananas are in season all-year round, and are dense in calories, making them a very important staple.

The amount of calories we want to eat in a day on a fruit-based diet is the same amount we would want to eat on any other diet: enough to sustain our activity levels. I will say though that it is darn near impossible to eat too many calories from fruit and vegetables. Unlike other foods that are heavily seasoned, or processed, or in some way altered to over-entice our taste buds, fruit will no longer be appealing once you are full. In fact, you will likely experience satiety like you never have before due to the fact that you are eating so much fiber and getting so many micronutrients and phytonutrients.

Mono-meals for optimum digestion, assimilation and energy: the less ingredients you have in a meal, the better it will digest and assimilate. For those people who are experiencing severe digestive issues, especially Crohn's disease and ulcerative colitis, this is especially important. The more ingredients in a single meal, the more work the body must do to break it down. So while not necessary to do all the time, mono-meals of one type of fruit are best, especially if you experience digestive problems.

Writing a primer on how to eat a fruit-based diet is one of those parts of the book that is almost painful to write. This is so incredibly simple that a lot of times I feel silly having to explain this to students and people who ask for help. Eating a fruit-based diet is simple, and there is no need to over complicate it. Here are a few simple guidelines:

- **The simpler the better.** One ingredient meals are optimum for taste, digestion, and assimilation. The more limited the number of ingredients, the easier the body can digest them. The less work the body is doing digesting complex combinations of ingredients, the more energy is freed up to work on healing.
- **Eat when you are hungry and stop when you are full.** If you are not hungry, don't eat! Learn to

be in touch with your body's natural hunger signals and heed them.

- **Eat with the seasons.** The fruit that is in season will rotate throughout the year. Eating with the seasons ensures highest quality, best taste, and most affordable prices.
- **Fruits have different densities in terms of water content and calorie content.** High-water fruit is best for breakfast. Eat your most calorically dense meal toward the middle of the day, when digestion is optimal.
- **Include leafy greens mostly during the last meal.** If you have nuts or seeds, eat them as part of the last meal as well.

Dr. Ben's Autoimmune Protocol

So how does this all break down into a meal plan you can implement in the real world? I'm going to lay out a basic structure. This is what I recommend doing, but of course, there is room for variability in terms of what types of fruits or vegetables are eaten at which meal times; however, this I believe is the most practical way to do this in the real world. A basic structure of what to eat in a day is as follows:

- **Breakfast:** Single-ingredient meal of high water fruit. Fruit will vary depending on seasonality. Right now in December 2020, I'm usually having papaya or pomegranate for my first meal because they are in season.

- **Lunch:** Banana smoothie with leafy greens. For an adult male, that is often a dozen bananas and half a head of lettuce or other leafy green. The bananas should be spotty-brown ripe. Green or yellow bananas will not blend or digest well, nor will they taste as good. For more green smoothie recipes and inspiration check out Dr. Ben's Green Smoothie Guide, free exclusively for book readers at http://bonus.createhealthbook.com

- **Dinner:** A small meal of fruit to start, followed by a large salad with at least one head of leafy greens, and all the other fruit and tender veggies (e.g., cucumber, bell pepper, etc.) you want. Also, include flax/hemp/chia seeds as desired. Both savory and sweet salad dressings can be made out of fruits, vegetables, and seeds. Visit my book bonuses page for more various homemade dressing recipes.

Salad Dressings

Simple Tahini Lemon

- 3 tbsp. of tahini

- Juice of 1 lemon or lime

This recipe can be easily whisked together with a fork.

Fancy Tahini Lemon

-3 tbsp tahini

-Juice of 1 lemon or lime

-1 minced clove of garlic

-1/2 minced bunch of parsley leaves

-1 date (soaked*)

Use blender or food processor

Applesauce Boss

Use as little water as possible. Finely dice the apples before blending.

- 3–4 medium apples

Optional: 1–2 RIPE pears

- Cinnamon to taste

Asian Dressing:

- 3 tbsp. tahini

- 3 dates (soaked)

- 1 cup fresh OJ

- 1 knuckle of ginger

Visit my book bonus resources page for more delicious dressing recipes. This protocol is simple but not easy. Later in the book we'll get into practical tips about how to do this consistently in the real world.

Sample Meal Plan by Season

Winter

Breakfast: Fresh squeezed orange 48–64 ounces (1.5–2 liters). I recommend getting a citrus press juice— they are the fastest and the easiest to clean. Optional: blend in basil.

Lunch: Green smoothie: 1.5–2 cups water; 8–12 bananas; ½ head of organic lettuce, spinach, or celery; plus 1–2 handfuls of frozen berries.

Dinner: Salad with 1–1.5 heads of lettuce, 1 bell pepper chopped, 1 pomegranate de-seeded, 1 handful of grapes, 1 handful of hemp seeds.

Dressing: Blend 1 pomegranate + 1 avocado.

Breakfast: Fresh squeezed grapefruit juice: 48–64 ounces (1.5–2 liters).

Lunch: Green smoothie:1.5–2 cups water; 8–12 bananas; ½ head of organic lettuce, spinach, or celery; plus 1 handful of grapes.

Dinner: Salad with 1–1.5 heads of lettuce, 1 cucumber + 1 tomato, 5–10 tangerines peeled and sectioned, 1–2 handfuls of grapes, 1 handful of hemp seeds.

Dressing: Blend 1 orange + 1 tomato + 1 avocado.

Breakfast: 1 large bowl of tangerines.

Lunch: Green smoothie: 1.5–2 cups water; 8–12 bananas; ½ head of organic lettuce, spinach, or celery; 4–6 soaked dates.

Dinner: Salad with 1–1.5 heads of lettuce, 1 bell pepper + 1 tomato chopped, 1 medium avocado chopped, 1–2 handfuls of grapes, 1 handful of hemp seeds.

Dressing: Juice of 1–2 lemons + 1–2 tablespoons of tahini, whisked into a suspension.

Spring

Breakfast: Large bowl of peaches and or nectarines.

Lunch: Green smoothie: 1.5–2 cups water, 7–10 bananas, ½ head of organic lettuce, 1 handful of blueberries, 1 handful of strawberries.

Dinner: Salad with 1–1.5 heads of lettuce, 1 bell pepper + 1 tomato chopped, 1 handful of blueberries, 2 handfuls of strawberries, 1 handful of hemp seeds.

Dressing: Blend 1–2 medium tomatoes + 1–2 mangos. Optional: pulse blend in cilantro.

Breakfast: Blended 1–3 mangos + 1–2 handfuls of berries over 1–2 mangos chopped.

Lunch: Green smoothie: 1.5–2 cups water, 6–9 bananas, ½ head of organic lettuce, and 2–3 mangos.

Dinner: Salad with 1–1.5 heads of lettuce, 1 cucumber chopped, 2–3 mangos diced, 1 handful of hemp seeds.

Dressing: Juice of 1–2 lemons + 1-2 tablespoons of tahini, whisked into a suspension.

Breakfast: Chop 2–3 peaches, blend 2–3 mangos, and pour over peaches.

Lunch: Green smoothie: 1.5–2 cups water, 8–12 bananas, ½ head of celery.

Dinner: Salad with 1–1.5 heads of lettuce, 2 bell peppers chopped, 1 mango + 1 peach diced. 1 handful of hemp seeds

Dressing: Blend 1 avocado + 1 tomato + 1 orange.

Summer

Breakfast: 1 medium or large watermelon. Blend or cut in half and eat with a spoon. Optional: squeeze lemon or lime on/in it as well.

Lunch: Green smoothie: 1.5–2 cups water, 8–12 bananas, ½ head of lettuce

Dinner: Salad with 1–1.5 heads of lettuce, 1 bell pepper chopped, 1 avocado sliced, 1 handful of hemp seeds.

Dressing: Blend 1–2 tomatoes + 1–2 mangos.

Breakfast: Chop 4–6 mangos. Enjoy with a fork!

Lunch: Green smoothie: 1.5–2 cups water, 5–8 bananas, ½ head of lettuce, 3–4 mangos.

Dinner: Salad with 1–1.5 heads of lettuce, 1 zucchini spiralized, 1 handful of hemp seeds.

Dressing: Blend 1 large avocado + 2 handfuls of grapes.

Breakfast: 1–3 honeydew or cantaloupe melons. Make sure they have ripened!

Lunch: Green smoothie: 1.5–2 cups water, 6–10 bananas, ½ head of lettuce, 1–2 handfuls of frozen berries.

Dinner: Salad with 1–1.5 heads of lettuce, 1 cucumber chopped, 2–3 handfuls of grapes and/or berries, 1 handful of hemp seeds.

Dressing: Blend 1 avocado + 3 stalks celery + 1 tomato + handful of dill.

Autumn

Breakfast: 1–3 pomegranates depending on size. Eat with a spoon.

Lunch: Green smoothie: 1.5–2 cups water, 8–12 bananas, ½ head of lettuce.

Dinner: Salad with 1–1.5 heads of lettuce, 1 tomato, and 1 bell pepper chopped; 2–3 handfuls of grapes, 1 handful of hemp seeds.

Dressing: Blend 1 avocado + 1 pomegranate.

Breakfast: 2–4 pounds of grapes, whole or blended.

Lunch: Green smoothie: 1.5–2 cups water, 5–10 bananas, ½ head of lettuce, 1–3 handfuls of grapes.

Dinner: Salad with 1–1.5 heads of lettuce, 1 zucchini spiralized, 2–3 handfuls of grapes, 1 handful of hemp seeds

Dressing: Blend 1 avocado + 1 tomato + 1 orange.

Breakfast: 250–500 grams (8-16oz) of dates, dry, soaked, or blended.

Lunch: Green smoothie: 1.5–2 cups water, 5–10 bananas, ½ head of lettuce, 5–10 soaked dates.

Dinner: Salad with 1–1.5 heads of lettuce, ½ cucumber diced, 2–3 handfuls of grapes, 1 handful of hemp seeds

Dressing: 1 avocado + 1 tomato + 1 orange blended

And remember, don't forget to pick up your free copy of Dr. Ben's Green Smoothie Guide free exclusively for book readers at http://bonus.createhealthbook.com

Practical Tips for Dr. Ben's Protocol.

Eating enough calories. The most common problem people encounter is not eating sufficient calories to sustain themselves. Fruits and vegetables are nutritionally dense but calorically poor. That is, on a nutrition plan of fruits and vegetables, a person needs to eat two to three times the volume or mass of a standard Western diet to get the same amount of calories. So most people are acclimated to eating way less food in terms of volume, but way more in terms of calories. This means it takes time to get used to eating much more volume in a sitting, in order to get sufficient calories.

You must develop a stretch in your stomach. In order to be able to get sufficient calories in a single meal, one needs to develop a stretch in one's stomach. The stomach, believe it or not, is made out of muscle tissue. It expands and contracts similar to your bicep or your hamstring. Most people rarely stretch out their stomach on a Western diet, because they don't need to when eating such calorically dense foods. The average person's stomach holds about one liter of volume. But to get enough calories in a single meal, one often needs to eat or drink two liters of food. It takes time to develop this stretch in one's stomach. My suggestion is to eat until you are full and then have one-to-two more bites of fruit or sips of a smoothie. Over time this builds a stretch in the stomach such that it can handle two liters of volume in a sitting. Until that time, one may need to eat five-to-six smaller meals throughout the day to get all the necessary calories until that stretch in the stomach is built. In general, it takes about two-to-three weeks to develop enough stretch in one's stomach to handle eating two liters of volume in a sitting.

Interesting side note. In my early twenties, I was once roommates with a semi-professional competitive eater. He had a whole regimen to build primary things: jaw strength/endurance and stretch in his stomach to handle more food. He would make giant batches of boiled cabbage, put salt on it, and eat it until his stomach could hold no more; then, continuously eat more as room opened up in his stomach, drinking tons of water to hold the stretch. He got to the point where he could hold five liters of food in his stomach. I don't recommend this kind of thing as healthy, but it was fascinating to see what the body was capable of when he pushed it. For most people, being able to stretch their stomach to two liters is plenty.

Grocery shopping, ripening, and storing. Eating a fruit-based diet requires a novel approach for shopping, as well as storing fruit in the home. The main challenges are the following:

1) Fruit is generally not ripe when you buy it from the store.

2) The ripening process is gradual and varies depending on the fruit.

3) The amount of time fruit stays at a peak ripeness where it is edible, but before it goes bad, is finite. The fruit must be eaten in this time frame, not before or after.

4) The amount of time a fruit stays ripe can be artificially prolonged by refrigerating it or freezing it.

5) As a consequence of one and two above, often we need to carry a lot of inventory in our home, in various stages of ripening to ensure we always have enough fruit to eat, but not too much that some is going bad. I tend to err on the side of the latter, just to ensure I always have adequate supply.

The best way to handle these challenges is to grocery shop twice a week, even if one of the trips is small, just to get a few things like bananas and greens. You will find yourself buying large quantities of a few things, rather than a mix-and-match variety of many things.

I also advise having some sort of storage system, such as a wood or metal set of shelves, to store the fruit and sort things by variety and by ripeness. You will always have fruit in various stages of ripening in the home, typically carrying about five-to-seven days' worth of inventory at any given time; otherwise, you may find yourself running out of fruit rather often and being unable to find ripe fruit that's ready to eat when you go to the grocery store.

Eating a fruit-based diet is definitely a manner of living that will require you to get accustomed to it. It takes time. But eventually you develop a system that keeps sufficient inventory in the home and requires very little conscious maintenance.

When and How to Reintroduce Cooked Food

At some point, you will likely not want to do a 100 percent raw fruit-based diet indefinitely. I know that I ate one for over three years because I feared that if I went back to cooked food, my disease symptoms would come back. The good news is that they did not! At some point along the way I had reversed my disease well enough that my body could tolerate some cooked, whole plant foods without issues. To determine how long that needs to be for you, at this point I don't have an answer. During the three-year period I had a major flare of eczema at about the one-year mark when I went through a relationship breakup after being symptom free for that entire year. I had no changes to my diet but that stressful situation re-triggered one (and only one) of my symptoms.

I would generally advise people to reintroduce cooked food on a limited basis, usually eaten with the dinner meal, after they have been symptom free for at least a few weeks or months. This definitely does not mean to cook all food or going back to the standard Western diet! This would be the reintroduction of cooked whole plant foods, such as steamed and roasted vegetables, gluten-free grains, and legumes . . . in limited quantities. The bulk of the diet should still be fresh fruits and vegetables. Processed food and animal foods will likely cause your symptoms again!

Here is a list of cooked foods that will generally not cause symptoms once you have reversed your condition:

- steamed greens
- sweet potatoes (steamed or bake)
- potatoes (steamed or bake)
- steamed cruciferous veggies (broccoli, cauliflower)
- gluten-free grains like rice, quinoa, millet and buckwheat
- legumes (ideally made from dried stock, soaked 24–48 hours, or longer, before cooking)

I would still recommend continuing to eat fruit-based for the first two meals of the day and including cooked plants with the dinner meal. If cooked food is reintroduced too soon, your symptoms may likely come back! Err on the side of waiting longer.

Chapter 6: The Mind-Body Connection and Why it Matters

This chapter is not intended to convince you of anything that conflicts with your existing beliefs. Let me tell you, as a former mechanical engineer, I used to scoff at anything "spiritual" or "woo-woo." I saw the world as purely material and mechanical. It was not until I had several firsthand spiritual experiences that showed me there was a world beyond the mechanical and material.

Most notably, I noticed that when I tried to change my diet and my lifestyle, many difficult emotions came up to be processed. When I could no longer suppress negative emotions with food, there was a lot of underlying baggage that needed to be sorted through.

I got into mind-body techniques, such as meditation, breathwork, tapping, and energy work, because there were problems that I simply could not solve through any other means. When it comes to mind-body techniques that I teach, it is not my intention to convince you of anything that conflicts with your existing beliefs. These techniques are simply tools that will work even if you don't believe in them. So leverage what's here.

I want to first start off by explaining the importance of the nervous system, then we'll dive more into the mind-body connection and my protocol for creating mental and emotional health.

Nervous System Modulates Immunity: Overview

Your nervous system is the most important system in your body because it is the master control system of every other system in your body. It controls not only your muscle movements but the actions of all your organs, tissues, and glands. If there is dysfunction in the nervous system, there will be downstream effects in any and possibly all systems in the body.

What many people fail to realize is that the nervous system even controls the immune system. Furthermore, through the works of brilliant scientists like biochemist Dr. Candace Pert (credited with the discovery of the opiate receptor, among many other discoveries), we now understand that the nervous system and the immune system are so intrinsically interlinked that it is difficult to separate one from the other and that many scientists call it a *neuroimmune system*, or the field of *neuroimmunology*. Ultimately, what's important here is that the nervous system has a pronounced effect on the immune system.

For instance, we know from laboratory experiments that white blood cells (a building block of our immune system) have been observed to transform into functional neurons (nervous system cells) in laboratory conditions. This is an intrinsic link that goes far beyond one system controlling the other.

But nervous system function modulates immunity. We know that if a person is exhausted or stressed out, their ability to fight infection is diminished. But it goes much more beyond that, as we'll get into here. Before we get more into that, I want to talk about some fundamental aspects of the nervous system you need to understand before we go deeper.

Autonomic Nervous System Overview

One of the fundamental components of the nervous system is the *autonomic nervous system*. This is the part of the nervous system that runs without any conscious thought. It handles all the functions that you don't consciously control, from your heart beating to your lungs breathing to your bowels moving and everything else you rarely, if ever, think about that is going on in your body.

The autonomic nervous system is broken down into two fundamental components that work opposite each other. There is the *sympathetic system*, also known as the "fight, flight, or freeze" system. This system kicks in when the body experiences a threat, whether that is imminent, acute danger, or mental and emotional wear and tear from continuous stress. The sympathetic system prioritizes the systems in the body that best equip the body to defend itself from a threat. This includes making the heart beat faster, pumping more blood to the muscles, and having the lungs take faster but shallower breaths. The sympathetic system also de-prioritizes systems that are *not* vital to handling imminent threats. This means that important systems such as digestion (which energy-wise is very metabolically expensive to operate) and immunity are down-regulated to preserve energy for fleeing or fighting.

Opposite to the sympathetic nervous system is the *parasympathetic nervous system*. The name is a bit of a misnomer because *para* means simply "runs alongside," which it does, but it performs, essentially, opposite functions to the sympathetic nervous system. The parasympathetic system is the "rest, digest, and heal" system. One way to remember the names is that parasympathetic system acts as a "parachute." The main functions of the parasympathetic system are to slow down the heart rate, slow down the breathing rate while increases breathing depth, up-regulate digestion, and up-regulate the immune system. The parasympathetic nervous system kicks in when the body-mind reaches a relaxed state.

Now the sympathetic system originally evolved for humans and their ancestors in a much different environment than we live in today. It evolved in an environment of scarcity, where humans were "hunted gatherers" i.e. we gathered much more than we hunted, and we were hunted by other predatory animals. The body needed a defense mechanism to help it when there was an imminent threat of danger. These threats were occasional but very acute when they happened.

Today we live in a different world. We are generally not afraid of when a predatory animal is going to threaten our life. Most people in the developed world do not live under threat of violence to their life on a regular basis. Times we are placed in grave, acute danger are few and far between. However, we still experience threats, just in different forms. In the twenty-first century, we are essentially "micro-dosed" with stressors all day long. These individual things may not seem like much when I list them, but their cumulative effect on our nervous system, and as a consequence on our overall well-being, is profound.

From the moment we wake up we are exposed to stressors. Even the fact that an alarm is waking us up instead of the sun is a stress on our nervous system. We wake up to pollutants in our air, our water, and our food. We are exposed to more radiation than ever from our wireless devices, Bluetooth, Wi-Fi, smart meters, and cell towers. The glowing rectangles we expose ourselves to throughout our day stress our brains from excess light exposure and our nervous system. Our jobs, our bosses, our teachers, our finances, our relationships, our commutes, the news, and social media all can act as low-level stressors each day, whose cumulative effects really add up. These put the nervous system into a chronic sympathetic or "fight or flight" state. It is so insidious and ubiquitous that most people do not notice or just accept it as a part of modern twenty-first-century life.

What does this do to us physiologically to be in this chronic sympathetic state? It means that our digestive system and our immune system are constantly down-regulated. Our ability to stay healthy is constantly compromised. The ubiquity of chronic disease is worse than ever. Digestive problems are so common that drug ads to address these problems are all over television. These problems have become so common, they are essentially accepted as normal.

How does this fit into the puzzle with autoimmunity? Well, a down-regulated immune system and a down-regulated digestive system are going to make it difficult to heal from autoimmune disease. After all, the immune system is a major player in the disease, and many folks with autoimmunity have digestive issues. Clinically, over the years, I have observed that people can get their diets really good for a long period of time, even eating all raw for years and still struggle with residual autoimmune symptoms because they are in sympathetic "fight, flight, or freeze" overdrive.

What causes this sympathetic overdrive?

1. Large exposures to chronic stressors.
2. Past trauma stored in the nervous system: physical, mental, emotional, chemical
3. Poor coping skills for stress and trauma

As mentioned, in the twenty-first century, we are exposed to a great deal of chronic stressors just through our environment and daily lives. The more we can do to mitigate this exposure, the more stress we can keep off of our nervous system. No one is expected to completely eliminate stress from their lives, but the more you can do within reason, the better results you will see in your life. Some of the best ways to reduce this stress are the following:

1. **Minimizing your exposure to EMFs.** This means keeping your phone on airplane mode when not using it, and turning off your Wi-Fi when not using it.

2. **Minimizing your exposure to pesticides.** This means buying as much organic as possible and sticking to the Environmental Working Group's "Clean 15" for conventional produce. Obviously it is not realistic for many people to eat 100% organic, and this list gives us an idea of what produce is most important to eat organic, and what can be eaten conventional, with a minimal pesticide toxicity burden.

3. **Minimize your work stress.** There are also ways of mitigating work stress, such as choosing a position that doesn't require overtime, living near work for a shorter commute, and working for a boss who treats you well. I realize for many people changing these things is not realistic, but if you have options, these are great ways to lower your chronic stress burden.

The subject of healing from past trauma certainly warrants its own chapter and probably its own book. Just as the body can only eliminate a certain amount of toxins in a given timeframe—and if that threshold is reached, the body stores the excess in various organs, including the connective tissue—the body-mind does the same thing with trauma. If the body-mind experiences overwhelming trauma in a short period of time, it cannot emotionally process all of it, so the excess is stored in the nervous system and connective tissue. I realize this is counter to mainstream psychology that trauma is stored in the body as opposed to in the brain. I highly recommend reading the book *The Body Keeps the Score* by Dr. Bessel van der Kolk. This stored trauma in our body continues to keep our nervous system dysregulated. Our body-mind goes on constant high alert, vigilant for another traumatic threat. In this chronic sympathetic defense state, the body-mind never gives itself time out to heal itself. Its chronic vigilance begins to wear itself down, and chronic disease is almost always a downstream effect of this.

How Do We Balance Out Our Autonomic Nervous System?

Most of us live in a chronic sympathetic "fight, flight, or freeze" state. Our nervous system is sympathetic dominant, and our parasympathetic system is barely online at all. There are ways to both down-regulate the sympathetic and up-regulate the parasympathetic to get us back into balance.

How to downregulate the sympathetic nervous system. As mentioned, there are many ways to lower our chronic stress exposure on a daily basis. But not all of these options are available to everyone all the time. You can only do the best you can with what you've got. Thankfully, there are other things you can do.

One of my favorite and most effective ways to down-regulate the sympathetic nervous system is through principled, specific chiropractic care. Normally regarded as a "treatment" for back pain, chiropractic is actually far more powerful than most people have been led to believe. Chiropractic's original intention was to remove interference to the nervous system to allow the body to function optimally and fully express its potential. Self-healing becomes a natural downstream consequence when interference to the body's natural self-healing mechanisms are removed. When there is adverse tension in the body, the spinal cord and its constituent nerves and nerve roots can become impinged or impeded, distorting the flow of information through the nervous system. Chiropractic seeks to normalize this adverse tension and allow the nervous system to communicate freely.

If you are going to seek out chiropractic care, I highly recommend seeing a principled, vitalistic chiropractor, whose goal is to remove nervous system interference. Many chiropractors seek simply to treat pain and disregard the big picture. There are over two-hundred chiropractic techniques. The one that I have found most congruent for me to both practice and receive regular care myself is called *Network Spinal*, or NS. NS uses light touches to work directly with the nervous system, queuing the body to release its own tension and bound energy, instead of forcing the tension out of the body.

There are many other healing modalities that work to down-regulate the body's sympathetic response, such as acupuncture, massage, cranial-sacral, reiki, and so on. It's important to find something that is most congruent with you.

The human body-mind has not yet evolved to be able to fully handle the stressors of the twenty-first-century world on its own. It is perfectly OK, and a very good idea, to seek outside help in mitigating this stress level.

How to up-regulate the parasympathetic nervous system. Equally if not more important than downregulating the sympathetic response, is to *up*-regulate the parasympathetic "rest, digest, and heal" response. This is what truly allows us to heal not only physically but mentally and emotionally as well. We spend so much time in a constant sympathetic "fight, flight, or freeze" state that we have almost forgotten what it feels like to be calm, relaxed, and peaceful unless it's under the influence of chemical substances such as drugs or alcohol.

The fundamental way to shift into a parasympathetic state is to take slow, controlled breaths. These slow controlled breaths are the hallmark of a rested, relaxed state and can actually "trick" the body-mind into going into a parasympathetic state. Once these slow controlled breaths begin, the heart rate begins to slow down, and other systems like digestion and the immune system that were considered "non-mission critical" in the sympathetic state can come back on line.

One of the best ways to put yourself into this parasympathetic state is through meditation and breathwork. By taking the time to put away all distractions and simply focus on your breath and your body and nothing else, you pave the way for your body-mind to enter a much more deeply relaxed state.

I highly recommend making this a daily practice. There are many forms of meditation and breathwork. Once again I'm fairly agnostic to the specific type or technique that people use, as long as they do it. Personally, I prefer Vipassana meditation and SRI (somato-respiratory integration) breathwork, but there are many techniques out there. Having it be a habit you can do every day is the most important thing. It is more effective to meditate for three minutes a day, than it is to meditate for twenty minutes twice a week. There is something about consistency that is very powerful.

I've created a library of guided meditations and visualizations for you to use on a pay-what-you-wish basis. These are designed not only to help you reach that deeply relaxing parasympathetic state but also to program your mind with success for creating health and reversing disease. You can visit the library here: www.drbenjaminbenulis.com/meditations.

Dr. Ben's Protocol for Creating More Mental and Emotional Health

If you are going to do my diet and lifestyle protocol for reversing disease, I highly recommend that you consider the mental and emotional components of your health. Even the best information in the world can't be applied correctly or consistently if our mind isn't right. I want to outline some fundamental things you can do to help create more mental and emotional health, which will help you succeed long term at creating physical health and reversing disease.

Get started with your why. Reading this book is one thing, but putting it into practice is another. As Stephen Covey (author of *The 7 Habits of Highly Effective People*) said, "To know and not to do, is really not to know." Let's do so some doing, so you can ensure some knowing. This a three-part exercise to understand your why, and you will spend about five minutes on each part.

Part One: Make a list of all the symptoms you are going through. Include, of course, the physical symptoms: chronic pain, digestive problems, skin issues, sensitivities, fatigue, and the like. Include the mental and emotional symptoms as well. These might even be a longer list than the physical. It can include things such as feeling like no one understands, feeling like you have an invisible disease, fearing that you'll never get well, fearing what happens if the disease gets worse, fearing they'll have to cut out one of your organs or glands. It may be a very long list. Don't leave anything out. Take full stock of how this conditions is effecting you emotionally. It's very easy to fire off the physical symptoms. But dig deep here: How is this really effecting you? Continue here and don't move on to part two until you've given this *at least* five minutes of thought.

Part Two: Now let's dive into just how this disease is affecting other areas of your life. Write this on a new sheet of paper and break it into four parts: your family/relationships, your work, your social life, and your overall satisfaction with life. How is this disease affecting all of those things? Is it causing a strain on the relationship with your family members or with your significant other (I definitely experienced both of those things)? Is it affecting your ability to do your job well, be a top performer, or run your own business? Is it affecting your willingness to go hang out with friends? Do you find yourself staying in, just because you're physical or emotionally not feeling well? If you're single, have you abandoned dating because your health is just so bad? Have friends gotten mad at you or distanced themselves from you because they perceive your behavior as anti-social? Do you feel alienated from your friends because of the disease? Make a list of all this stuff. When you really take inventory here, you may find that your health is really impacting your life, even more negatively than you had assumed. That's OK. We're digging into this and putting all those cards out on the table for a reason. So make sure all the cards are out on the table before moving on to the next part.

Part Three: Congratulations, you put in the work in parts one and two, and this part will be a lot more fun. Now we want to look at how your life will change when you get well. What will be different? How will your relationships change? How will your social life change? What activities will you begin doing again, or what new ones will you try out? What are some things you've always wanted to do but felt you couldn't because your health was holding you back? Assume you'll have perfect health. What would you do if you knew there was no way your body, your mind, or your self-doubt could hold you back?

This list is critically important because it creates a clear picture of where we want to go. This is the kind of thing that is great to create a vision board around if you are so inclined. Often it can be way too easy to get caught up in the day-to-day to see the big picture. We know we're suffering with our health, but after a while we can learn to just live with it. But that is usually an unfulfilled life, absent of many things we'd like to be able to do, but we can't because of our health. If we can get clear on creating a compelling picture to work toward, it's much easier to stay motivated with the lifestyle and diet changes we know we need to make. People are in general much more motivated to move toward pleasure than they are away from pain. This allows us to get a clear picture of what we want, instead of constantly focusing on what we *don't* want, and that is much more motivating than just trying to avoid pain and the difficulties of the present circumstances.

So take this list of how your life will be different and post copies of it all throughout your home. Include pictures if you want. Post it on your fridge, on your bathroom mirror, on your bedroom mirror, all the places you know will see it. This will be a daily reminder of why you are doing what you are doing. Moving toward pleasure is a far stronger motivator than just avoiding pain. And many people are so encompassed in the pain and discomfort of the present, they never take the time to imagine how life could be better. With that end in mind, it is much easier to reach your destination.

Daily Habits to Create Mental and Emotional Health

1. I recommend meditating, praying, or doing breathwork twice a day for at least five minutes each time—once upon waking and once in the early afternoon. You can use the meditations in my free library or do what you like. If you have a religious faith, or a specific spiritual practice you adhere to, commit to doing that twice a day. I find that meditating for just five minutes twice per day is extremely powerful and confers much more benefit that meditating for longer but sporadically.

2. When you are struggling with difficult emotions, journal them. List out everything you are feeling. Some people call this a "brain dump." Get out on paper any and all thoughts, feelings, and emotions that you are experiencing, and you will find that they will weigh significantly less on your mind.

3. Getting adequate sleep is critical. I recommend setting a bedtime of 9 p.m., or 10 p.m. at the latest, and shutting off all electronics an hour before that

bedtime. Getting adequate sleep is critical for both mental and emotional health.

4. Spend time outside each day, at least ten minutes, ideally in nature if you can't.

5. Have at least one person in your life you can be completely radically honest with: someone who you can tell exactly what you're thinking, feeling, and experiencing without judgment. This can be a family member, friend, or partner. Having this channel of communication is extremely important for being able to express things that are troubling you.

Chapter 7: How to Succeed in the Real World

This chapter is all about how to apply everything I've taught and succeed at it in the real world. The real world is *not* set up for you to be well, where disease is the default state. Just look at the various food options when you drive down any given street. To overcome the status quo and build new healthy habits, it will take work and a whole lot of mistakes along the way. This is a primer on how to succeed for the long haul.

Finding the best deals on produce

Let's face it, shopping for tons of produce, especially organic produce, can get expensive. If there are ways you can reduce the cost, you want to do it. Foraging is just one of many ways, but definitely not an option for everyone.

One thing I recommend is pulling up pricing on the internet before you go shopping. This way you can price-compare and always get the best deals. I recommend doing this by finding all of the grocery stores in your area, pulling up their weekly sale website and bookmarking it in a folder. Call the folder something like "Weekly Deals." Then, each week when you're planning your food shopping, you can open all the deals in that folder in a new browser window, in separate tabs. This will allow you to window shop from the comfort of your own home and know which grocery stores have the best deals.

If you can find a produce wholesaler in your area, that is another great option. Since they typically don't sell direct to consumer, they can often be a little hard to find. You may have to do some internet sleuthing to find one, or ask grocery stores and restaurants where they get their produce. If you can find an organic one, even better. You may also have to negotiate with them to even have them let you buy from them. Often they will say they only sell to other businesses. If you let them know you will be paying cash, and you're willing to buy by the case, often they'll be willing to sell. When I lived in Los Angeles, I bought from wholesalers all the time and got amazing deals. Often, if they have produce that is too ripe to sell but perfect to eat, they will sell it to you at a steep discount because they can't sell it to another business.

Another place you can often buy in bulk is farmer's markets. If you are willing to buy fruit or vegetables in bulk, they will give you a better price. And just like wholesalers, they will also be willing to cut you a deal on "seconds" produce that is getting a little too ripe or has blemishes on it. I also like farmer's markets because if you shop there every week, you can often build relationships with your farmers where they will let you in on the best of their crop, get first pick at new stuff, and often be cut deals just for being a regular customer.

Foraging

Foraging is the act of picking fruit from trees growing in the wild, or in your neighborhood. If you are fortunate to live in an area where fruit grows, foraging can be a fun health-promoting hobby and a great way to get free top-quality fruit. I have lived in Los Angeles, Berkeley, and Phoenix, and I foraged lots of fruit in all of these areas. This may not be available in your area, but many people have more fruit growing where they live than they think, they just have to go out and try to find it.

Available fruit will change with the seasons, so there is always something new to forage:

December–March: oranges, grapefruit

December–January: dragon fruit

April/May (later in more northern climates): mulberries, loquats

Summer: wild blueberries

August–October: figs

September–November: dates

September–November: guava

September–December: pomegranates

Understand that the vast majority of people who have fruit trees on their property never pick the fruit, or at least no more than a few pieces of fruit. In my experience, when you knock on their door and ask to pick from their tree, they almost always say yes. And if they do say no, they're usually super polite about it. So actual confrontation is rare; most people are super friendly. Bring your own box and load up!

If you are looking to forage in your own area and find people who have trees that are willing to let you pick, there are two websites that I highly recommend using. The first is called www.fallingfruit.org: this is a user-generated map of fruit trees in your area. You can find trees that other people have marked, as well as mark your own. Understand that even though the trees are there, the fruit will only be there if it's in season. You can mark which ones are on public property and can be picked and which ones are on private property and need permission.

Another website I recommend using is Nextdoor. This allows you to communicate with people in your immediate neighborhood. Sometimes you can actually find people giving fruit away. But what it's most useful for is posting want ads to pick. You can say something like "Does anyone have any mulberry trees that are dropping tons of fruit right now? Don't let them stain your car and your driveway. I'll come pick them!" Often times if you frame it in terms of your helping them, they are even more likely to say yes.

When picking from someone else's tree, it's super important to be polite, respectful, and thankful to them afterward. People are usually wary of letting strangers on their property, even if it's to pick fruit that they'll never use. The more pleasant an experience you make it for them, the more likely you are to be able to come back another time or next year to pick again.

I recommend keeping some kind of personal Word document or spreadsheet of all the available fruit trees in your area. That way you can go back year after year and pick from the same spots. I'm now at a place where during the citrus season and mulberry season, I literally know of so many trees; I can never run out of fruit to pick during these times.

Cravings

When you make big changes to your diet, it's almost inevitable that you will experience cravings for the old foods that no longer serve you. These foods that are often laden with salt, refined sugar, and refined oil are in their nature addictive. Concentrated sources of calories rarely occur in nature, so our brain is programmed to seek them out. The problem is that these refined foods may be super concentrated in calories but, in doing so, have removed almost all the nutrition. So, as an unfortunate side effect, the more refined the food is, the more addictive it is.

Dairy products are particularly addictive and were the most difficult for me to quit. Many people share this sentiment. Dairy products have compounds in them that when broken down in the digestive tract turn into what's called *casomorphins*, which are essentially opioid-analogs that create an opiate-like effect. So cheese is literally chemically addictive. It is probably one of the hardest food addictions to break.

So if you get cravings for these things, what is the best way to handle it?

Dr. Ben's Top Tips for Preventing Cravings

1. Make sure you are eating enough. I think this is the number one cause for most cravings. Since fruits and vegetables have so few calories, you can eat a *ton* of volume and still not consume very many calories. So you have to get used to eating *a lot* of fruits and vegetables to stay satiated. This may mean eating more small meals throughout the day in the beginning to build the stretch in your stomach. Over time, you'll be able to fit bigger meals in and need to eat less frequently to get sufficient calories.

2. If you go to an event where there will be food, eat beforehand *and* bring your own. This ensures that you have something to eat so your brain doesn't rationalize "there was no food there I could eat!" Always be prepared. It is no one else's responsibility to feed you healthy food or to take care of your health

other than you. Being willing to take responsibility for your health is huge. If you want to reverse disease, your health is in your own hands, not anyone else's.

3. Regular daily meditation (*not* when cravings are hitting). Let me explain why this helps so much. It can be very difficult to stop and slow down in the throes of a craving and sit with the feeling. Often, sometimes we are so uncomfortable, stressed, or anxious that we see the food we crave as an escape to these bad feelings. And since processed, calorie-dense foods numb your feelings, it becomes an easy path for escape. But if you've been meditating regularly, this process becomes easier. Slow down. Sit with it. Listen to your body. Try to understand what you are craving and why. Are you truly hungry? Or is this an attempt to suppress emotions with food? If you have a regular meditation practice, it becomes much easier to do this. Because for people who meditate regularly, their thoughts are less in control of them than most people. It can be very easy to let unconscious programming steer the ship, especially in times of stress. Meditation allows you to have more conscious awareness over your own thoughts so that they're not steering the ship.

OK but—what about when those cravings actually hit? You've done your best to prevent them using the three tips above. But those calorically dense animal or processed foods are just getting the best of you. What do you do?

Dr. Ben's Top Tips for Addressing Cravings When They Happen

1) As uncomfortable as this sounds, sit with it. As much as you probably want to jump out of your own skin in the moment, just sit with it and take some deep breaths in through the nose and out through the mouth. Do not attempt to "resist" the craving. Just listen to it. Ask yourself, What does my body want? Why am I feeling this way? What is coming up for me? There are no right or wrong answers to these questions. But the act of checking in can be very calming. Often times we have alienated or repressed parts of ourselves that we have not listened to in a long time. By giving these emotions that come up space to be expressed, it can often lessen or eliminate the craving considerably.

2) Use an exercise that is called Emotional Freedom Technique, or "Tapping." This is a body-mind technique based on tapping on the different acupuncture points to calm the nervous system. Often during a craving, our hindbrain, the survival-fight-or-flight mechanism of our nervous system is triggered. It becomes very difficult to think clearly or act rationally. Tapping overrides that and calms down the amygdala. Best of all, it's free; it requires no equipment, and you can do it immediately. For a tutorial on tapping, visit: http://www.drbenjaminbenulis.com/eft-tapping-for-cravings.

3) If the craving still persists, compromise with a slightly less healthy food. I sometimes call this practice *bailing*, which is a term from extreme sports where one "bails" on a difficult trick and does a much easier trick instead of falling over, or not doing a trick at all. Instead of French fries or pizza, make some simple cooked plant foods, such as a steamed sweet potato with steamed greens. This can satisfy the cravings for warm, cooked foods without seriously disrupting the detoxification and healing processes.

OK so hopefully you've been able to stave that sucker off. But what if you haven't? What if you screwed up and ate pizza or French fries or whatever crazy food you just had to have. What do you do then? Well I'm certainly not going to leave you in the lurches and tell you "too bad, you suck!" Because to be perfectly honest . . . this happens to everyone, especially in the beginning. I had absolutely *none* of these coping skills in the beginning. I was doing this totally on my own in the beginning, with *zero* supportive friends. So I had quite a few instances where I gave into cravings. And—Wow!—my body let me know it didn't like that. So you've given in to the craving, now what?

1) If you give in to the craving, understand that *it happens to the best of us.* Do not beat yourself up. Like riding a bike, dust yourself off and jump back on. Is it possible you may "pay" in terms of symptoms coming back? Absolutely. See this as a good sign. It

means that your body is communicating to you what it likes and what it doesn't like. As you go further down this path, it narrows. And the price for veering off in terms of symptoms often becomes more severe. Over time, it just doesn't even feel worth it anymore to eat unhealthy because of how bad your body will react.

2) Don't use one fall off the horse as an excuse to go on a bender of several meals of this stuff. Have your one mistake, acknowledge it, *forgive yourself*, and move on. It can be very tempting to fall off the bike on a Saturday and go, "Monday I'll get back on it," and take Sunday to just completely destroy yourself with unhealthy foods. Backsliding that far is much harder to recover from. Get back on it the very next meal. Often times, the best thing can be to prepare that next meal, even if it's breakfast the next day and have it ready to go.

3) Do not use words like "good" or "bad" to describe how you ate. You are not a five-year-old who needs to be punished for bad behavior. You can use the words "I was compliant" or "I stayed on the program," instead of "I was not compliant" or "I veered off the program." Eating unhealthy does *not* make you a bad person, so stop calling unhealthy eating *bad* behavior. And conversely, eating healthy does not make you a good person. I've met plenty of people who eat really healthy who are not good people! There is no correlation, so stop saying "I was good today" or "I was bad today" when it comes to eating.

If you cut someone off in traffic today, you were bad, but if you ate half-a-dozen donuts in the parking lot in one sitting, you were just noncompliant. You are not a five-year-old. Stop calling yourself "bad" for making poor eating choices, seriously.

4) Most importantly, move on and don't dwell. If it happened yesterday, it's in the past now, and there's absolutely no reason to beat yourself up or to dwell on it. The present moment is new, and you can make new choices. If you are beating yourself up about noncompliant choices you made yesterday or last week, you are not serving yourself. So just forgive yourself, forget it, and move on. The present moment is always the best time to start over fresh.

How to Handle When You Do Slipup

First off, let me say this: There will be slipups. I have not met anyone who made the decision to radically change their diet, did it, never looked back, and never slid back. It happens to *everyone*. And believe me, it happened to me. I can definitely remember in 2012 puking in the bushes after a friend offered me a few Oreos and I didn't refuse. That was one of many incidents. I didn't really have a support system back then, it was just me. So there was *a lot* of two steps forward one step back. But guess what, that is still one net step forward.

The key thing here is not how bad you slipup but how often you slip and what you eat when you slip. The keys to getting back on the right track are the following:

1. **How quickly you nip the slipup in the bud.** The quicker the turn around on that, the easier it gets. If the slipup turns into a protracted, multiday binge, it's a lot easier to rationalize continuing than it is to turn it around. So the sooner you can turn it around, the easier it is to do so. If you're in the middle of a longer bender, it may be more work, but it's definitely necessary work.

2. **How you talk to yourself about it.** If you are negative and beat yourself up, it's going to be a lot harder. But if you stay positive, are able to forgive yourself, and move on, it makes it much easier. If you use phrases like "I was bad" or "I was good," that will slow your progress. You're not a five-year-old. You're an adult. There's no going to a timeout for "being bad." Either you stayed on protocol, or you went off protocol. But how healthy you eat does not determine your worth as a person. So don't use words that allow what you eat to define you as a person. It is only your actions we are concerned with, and they are either compliant—or they aren't. That's a very important distinction.

3. **Don't dwell on your mistakes.** Get back on protocol and don't look back. By making a mistake, you just learned something, how you can be more successful next time. See the mistake as a lesson you can

use going forward, instead of dwelling on it. Instead of having a win-lose mentality, where you can either win or lose, have a win-learn mentality, where you can either win or you can learn something when you don't.

Handling Social Situations

This is probably something that people fear the most. In Western society, we put so much emphasis on food being a part of social gatherings. We create community by giving each other food or cooking for each other. It is an act of love, and act of service to provide someone else food. So when you come along and say, "No, thank you, I'm on a wellness program to reverse my ankylosing spondylitis," prepare to get some weird stares. For many people, the thought of sticking out or being called out because of your eating is about as frightening as public speaking, which many people rate scarier than death.

Here are some basic strategies and tips that will make this kind of thing a lot easier:

1. **Eat before you go.** Fill up on a smoothie or a big salad before you go. It will make temptation much easier resist, and you can say with confidence "no thanks, I ate before I got here"

2. **Bring your own (BYO).** I can't stress this enough: *always* BYO. I find the best thing is to bring a Tupperware container with a giant salad and another

Tupperware container full of fruit. Bring more than you could possibly eat all by yourself. That way there is plenty to share. It's much easier to disarm questions if you have plenty of extra to offer others. It allows you to fit in socially more if you're sharing the food that you brought. So take the time to make a lot of something really good and bring it!

3. **Doctor's orders.** If anyone asks why you're refusing food or eating your own food, you can always play the doctor card: "I'm working with a doctor who specializes in helping a condition I have, and this is what he wants me eating. It's the only way I'm going to be able to [get off this nasty medication/be able to walk normally again/avoid having my colon cut out/ etc.]." Generally, people will leave you alone after hearing this kind of thing.

4. **Carry yourself with calm confidence.** People will pick up on how you carry and present yourself. If you seem defensive or unsure of yourself or timid, they may be more likely to criticize, question, or persecute. But if you act like it's no big deal, it's normal to eat fruits and vegetables, it's fun and enjoyable to eat fruits and vegetables; they are much more likely to go along with that sentiment and leave you alone. So don't get defensive. Remain calm and confident, and act like it's an everyday normal thing. After all, even if it isn't, I think we can agree it definitely should be!

How to Handle Travelling

Travelling is one that trips a lot of people up, especially if they're travelling by airplane. How do you eat healthy and stick to this program when you're on the road? Well, the answer is pretty much the same way you do when you're at home or you're at work: you just plan ahead a lot better.

1. **Bring a lot of produce with you.** Even if you arrive in a new city, you can go to the grocery store there, but for the most part, the fruit they have there won't be ripe. And you don't want to be stuck without ripe fruit. So the best way to do that is to pack a forty-pound banana box full of ripe fruit, and include your blender in that box too if need be. The best part about these boxes is that they fit conveniently in the overhead bin of an aircraft. I'll never forget the time I was interviewed by a guy named Robert Gruler on his podcast; the first time he ever saw me, we were both flying from Phoenix to Orlando for a seminar, and I was carrying a giant box of fruit on the plane and loading it into the overhead bin. He told me he thought, "Who the hell is this guy, bringing a giant box of fruit on the plane? It's Florida, they'll have bananas there!"

2. **Scope out where to shop ahead of time.** Use a map service like Google Maps to find grocery stores that are nearby to where you're staying. Have your go-to spots planned out when you get there so that

you're not scrambling to find produce among all the other things you have to do once you land.

3. **Ask friends or family your visiting to shop for you.** If you are visiting friends or family, ask them to pick some things up for you ahead of time and offer to pay them back. This way you have produce waiting for you when you get there, one less thing to do when you arrive. And if you're dependent on other people for transportation while you're staying there, well that's one less trip someone has to take you on while you're staying.

If you coordinate these things ahead of time, it will be very easy to continue your diet as you normally do while you're travelling. *And*, it will probably save you a lot of money because it can be very easy to blow money on restaurant and hotel food while you're travelling.

How to Cultivate a Mindset for Success

In order to succeed at creating enough health to reverse a chronic autoimmune disease, just knowing what to do is not often enough. We live in a world now where the default state is dis-ease, a severe lack of health. The world is set up for you to be fat, sick, and miserable. There aren't health-food stores, fruit orchards, and gardens on every corner. Instead, there is McDonald's, Applebee's, KFC, and Fatburger. It's set up to make the most money, and unfortunately, getting you sick makes the most money. If you want to sidestep all of that and succeed at creating health, you are going to have to do most or all of it yourself.

One of the most important things to do is to get clear on your *why*. Why do you actually want to get well? Many people are content to stay sick and continue to feed their disease day after day. After all, it's not killing them, at least not any time soon. To them, creating health is just not worth the hassle. In their opinion, staying sick may not be fun, but it's way easier than working to create health.

In my years of doing this, I've noticed that the longer people go down the road of staying sick, eventually they hit some sort of breaking point. They get to a point where they can no longer tolerate how their disease is interfering with their life. It is more than just symptoms at this point. The disease and its symptoms are getting in the way of something that's important to them. It could be advancing in their career. It could be a hobby they love that they can no longer do. It could be playing with their kids or grandkids. It could just be wanting to be a healthy example for their kids, because they don't want what's happened to them to happen to their kids.

Eventually, people hit a point that Tony Robbins calls the *emotional leverage* point. This is the point where staying the same becomes actually more painful than changing. This is, of course, a perceived sense of painfulness. But it has just gotten too painful to continue on the way they are, and changing their diet and lifestyle habits, as difficult as that may seem, finally isn't as horrifying as continuing down the road they're on. I remember when I hit that point: waking up with a hangover, a throbbing headache, my muscles cramped throughout my whole body, and a horrible stomach ache, surrounded by my own vomit. I remember that day well, thinking, "Wow, something has to change, I can't keep living like this."

If you're reading this book, you probably have already hit this emotional leverage point, or at least come close. You're ready for a change, or you've finally admitted to yourself that it's the best path forward. It's important now to get clear on your why, and break it down into three parts. Because hitting that emotional leverage point is one thing, but harnessing the strength of that and maintaining it, even when things get tough, is another. Refer back to the previous chapter for my protocol on creating mental and emotional health.

How to Overcome Perfectionism

Do you struggle with perfectionism? No? OK, well, for the one person out there who does, I'm writing this for you, because literally no one else has that problem. But I know you would read this book, so I put this in here for you—yes just you. Because you're seriously the only one. Aren't you glad I wrote this one section specifically just for you?

Alright, the last paragraph was a joke because so many people struggle with this. So don't feel like you're alone. People want to believe that if they get their diet perfect or their morning routine perfect or their exercise program perfect or some aspect of themselves or their habits "perfect," that somehow it will magically change things.

This is what's called an *arrival fallacy*: somehow once perfection is achieved, results will magically arrive. Fortunately, it doesn't work like that. Results are built over time. And during that time of building new habits, mistakes will happen. Perfection is rarely if ever achieved. The good news is, results don't wait for those who are perfect. Results come to those who take action. And many people use their "perfectionism" as a way to delay (often indefinitely) taking action.

- "When things settle down at work, then I'll finally be ready to do Dr. Ben's program"
- "When the new year hits, I'll be magically blessed with a lot more free time to focus on taking care of my health"
- "After my kids get a little older, I'll have time to really dial in my diet and my health"

All of these follow a similar pattern of thinking. Once [outside condition] is satisfied then I'll finally be able to do [lifestyle change] well enough to succeed. Let me tell you that this perfectionist pattern of thinking is a recipe for **never taking action**. There will always be barriers in your life. The timing will never be perfect. The outside conditions will never be perfect. Your kids, your significant other, your job, your parents, none of that will ever just escort itself out of your way so you can focus 100 percent of your attention on your health and not make any mistakes. It's *not* going to happen. Let go of the fantasy. Instead start taking action with the resources and the time that you have and start learning by making mistakes, and in three months, six months, a year from now, you'll be really glad you started today and didn't wait.

How to Overcome Self-Criticism

This one is for all my fellow self-critics out there, for the people that no matter how good of a job they do, there is always an inner critic inside that can find *some* kind of fault. Let me first just tell you that I feel you on this. Even though I'm a lot better than I used to be, I still struggle with this aspect of things. So let me tell you a little bit about some tactics that have helped me.

Take imperfect action. Imperfect action is about ten times better than no action. Face it, you are going to make mistakes at some point, so might as well just get them out of the way early. Go in there with the understanding that despite your best efforts, you could be an absolute disaster. Oh well, too bad. Remember that "Every Master was once a Disaster."

Patronize your inner critic. When your inner critic chimes in and decides to give you some criticism about something that didn't go 100 percent perfectly, don't fight them or ignore them, just reply, "Thank you for sharing!" Say in it a serious tone, or a sarcastic tone, whichever feels right to you in the moment. Just acknowledge it and move on. Bonus points if you say, "Thank you for sharing!" out loud. Patronizing your inner critic instead of ignoring or fighting them is a great way to train yourself that that critical voice doesn't have power over you.

Praise yourself for your successes, even if they are super small. Did you drink a smoothie even though you were really jonesing for a burrito today? Give yourself a high-five or put on some music and do a little dance. Celebrate the small wins! Forge a new neural pathway that praises success instead of only having one that punishes failure. Success breeds success, and small wins breed big wins. So celebrate small wins!

By the way, junk food is not a way of actually "celebrating" any sort of win, whether it has to do with your health or otherwise. Food is not a reward unless you're a dog. There are plenty of other ways to reward yourself that don't involve self-harm.

Here are some of my favorites:

List of Ways to Reward Yourself (without food)

- Go for a walk in a secluded nature spot
- Book a visit to a trampoline park and bounce around
- Go out to a comedy club (two drink minimum can still be water)
- Volunteer at an animal shelter and play with the dogs
- Sign up for music lessons to learn an instrument
- Go see an afternoon movie when the theater isn't full (and sneak in bananas)
- Visit a new museum (and do a web search for free museum days)

- Teach yourself a new song on a musical instrument (from the internet)
- Sign up for classes or lessons on a new skill you want to learn

Final Word. It is my sincere hope that you found this book informative, entertaining, and enlightening, and I hope that I challenged your existing beliefs and thought processes on at least one subject. I hope that you are able to put what's here to use and make amazing things happen. I feel so blessed to be able to have shared this with you, and I hope the value that you get out of this book far exceeds whatever nominal price you paid for it.

ABOUT THE AUTHOR

Dr. Ben has been helping people heal from chronic disease and autoimmune conditions for nearly a decade. He holds a BSE in Mechanical Engineering from the University of Pennsylvania and worked for 10 years in the tech industry before coming down a with an autoimmune condition that doctors could neither diagnose nor treat. Forced to figure things out on his own he began to massively self educate and massively self experiment. Eventually healed himself with diet and lifestyle and now uses those experiences as the basis for what he teaches. He holds a Doctor of Chiropractic degree from the Los Angeles College of Chiropractic. He also completed a clinical preceptorship at the True North Health Clinic in Santa Rosa, CA which focused on healing chronic disease through healthy diet and supervised fasting. He now lives and practices in Phoenix, AZ where he also enjoys hiking, fruit foraging, road trips, strength training and performing stand up comedy.

Get free book bonuses and healthy recipes on his book bonus page here:

bonus.CreateHealthBook.com

Made in the USA
Coppell, TX
10 June 2022

78707684R00100